Fitness and Health with Nutrition

What is fitness?

"Fitness" is a broad term that means something different to each person, but it refers to your own optimal health and overall well-being. Being fit not only means physical health, but emotional and mental health, too. It defines every aspect of your health. Smart eating and active living are fundamental to fitness.

Fitness includes five essential components, flexibility, cardiorespiratory fitness, muscular endurance, muscular strength, and body composition. Fitness is vitally important to health and wellness as well as to the ability to engage in normal activities of daily living (ADLs) without excessive fatigue. Physical activity and exercise training programs should be designed with the intent of improving each of the key components of health-related physical fitness in addition to preventing chronic disease (e.g., heart disease, diabetes, osteoporosis etc.)

Fitness is a very personal term! Fitness is having a healthy mind, body, and spirit to allow you to maximize your potential and help others maximize their potential. Your definition of fitness will be influenced by your interests, physical abilities, and goals.

Being physically fit and healthy involves having a fit:

1. Mind
2. Body
3. Spirit

Fitness is the ability to function efficiently in an active environment that suits your personal interests and goals. You should have your own unique definition and create a baseline that you can build on throughout your life.

Your fitness goals should always be realistic and something you look forward to as part of your active lifestyle. Whether it's running a marathon or taking a walk, always operate in an environment that you can manage.

Functional fitness refers to how well you're able to do all the physical tasks you need to do each day. For example, if you're functionally fit, you can carry a bag of groceries without strain, bend down to pick up laundry from the floor without pulling a muscle, lift a child without injuring your back or even perform regular exercise. A large factor in functional fitness is flexibility - and staying active can help. Movement helps loosen up the body, keeping muscles limber.

Top 10 fitness exercises to do at home

Did you know that on your fitness journey it is just as important to focus on nutrition as well as intensive training? Here, as often in life, it comes down to the right balance. Do you want to build more muscles? Try to implement more protein into your diet. In addition to the classic protein sources like eggs, quark and meat, you can also try and include plant-based options like beans, soy or pseudo-grains like quinoa! If you want to lose weight, you need to be in a caloric deficit. It is not for nothing that they say, "Abs are made in the kitchen". However, it is important to go slow if your goal is losing weight. While dieting can often lead to quick weight loss, a lot of the time you risk putting on extra weight due to the so called "yo-yo effect".

Today we will show you 10 exercises that you can do at home and for which you don't need any equipment at all! We have 10 full body exercises for you, which focus on muscle building and definition.

1. HIGH KNEES
Intermediate

FITNESS, HEALTH, AND NUTRITION

Table of Contents

Abs, Quads, Arms

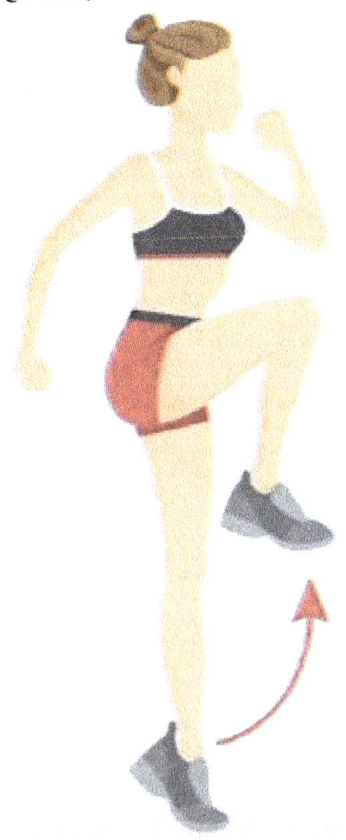

An exercise to get you going!
Stand shoulder width apart on your mat. Lift your right leg up.
Meanwhile, raise your right hand above your head and then
bring it in front of your body. The right hand should now meet
the right knee. Now put your leg back down and repeat the
process on the left side. Adjust the pace to whatever suits you
best. The faster you get, the more effective it will be!

2. SQUAT JUMPS
Beginner
Quads, Glutes

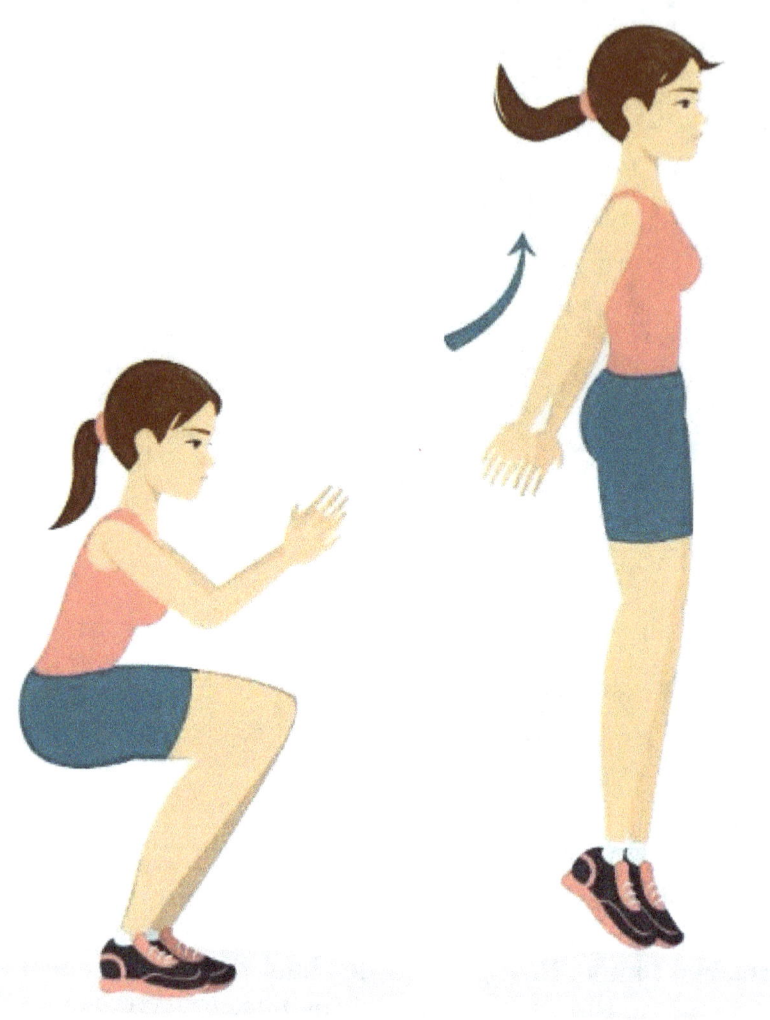

You will definitely work up a god sweat here!
Squat jumps are a popular warm-up exercise and easy to do as
well. Stand wide on your mat. Get into a squat position. Put
your hands in front of your body, keep your back straight,
bend your knees and squat down. Now jump out of the squat
as high as you can. Land in a squat position. Repeat this
process for about 30s – if you are more advanced, you can do
the exercise longer!

Note: Do not arch your back and always keep your knees behind your toes!

3. PUSH – UPS
Advanced
Shoulders, Arms, Upper Back, Abs

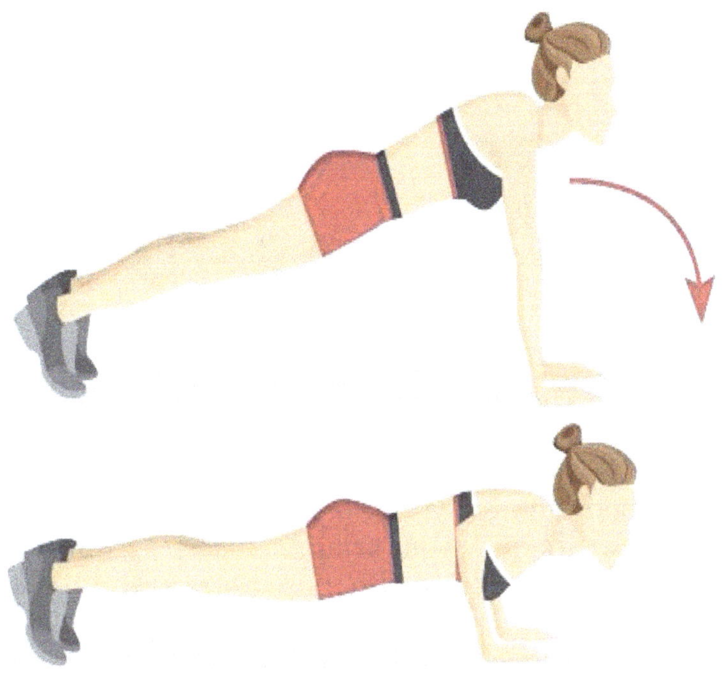

An incredible all-rounder exercise!
Lie flat on your stomach, position your hands under your shoulders and push yourself away from the floor, keep your body under tension! Look down. Your body should form a straight line. If this exercise is too difficult for you, you can keep your knees on the floor and try a simplified variation.
Note: Don't let your body sag, always keep tension!

4. SUPERMAN
Beginner
Back

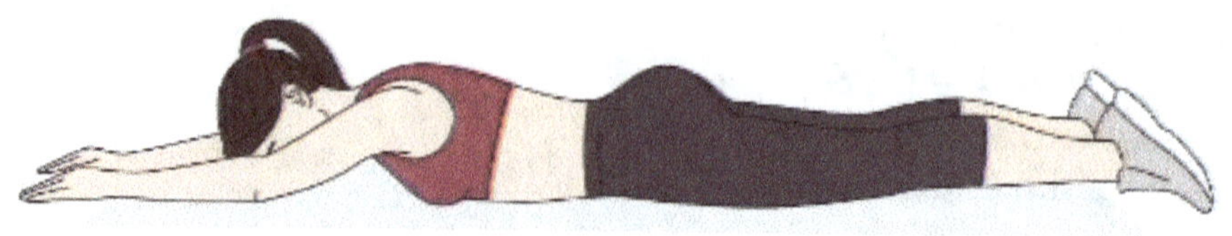

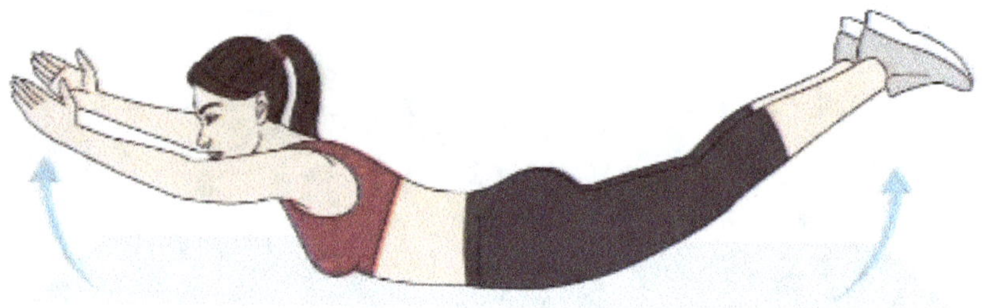

A beautiful rear can also endear!
This exercise is super easy and good for your back. Lie on your
stomach. Extend your arms forward. Look down. Now you pull
your upper body and your legs up. Hold the position for a few
seconds before dropping your arms and legs back onto the
mat. Try to move your body with muscle strength and not with
momentum!
Note: keep tension!

5. SIT–UPS
Intermediate
Abdominal muscles

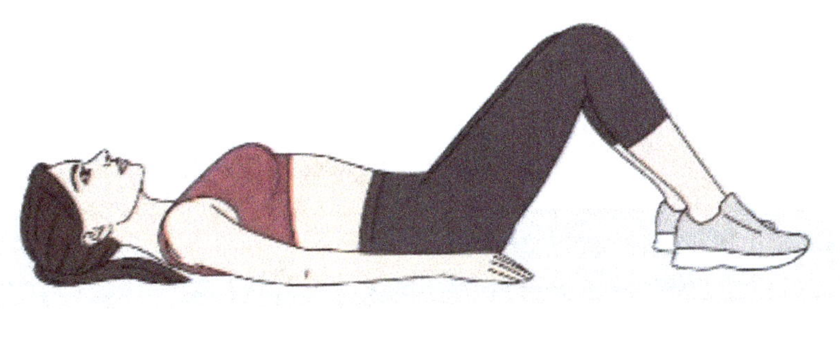

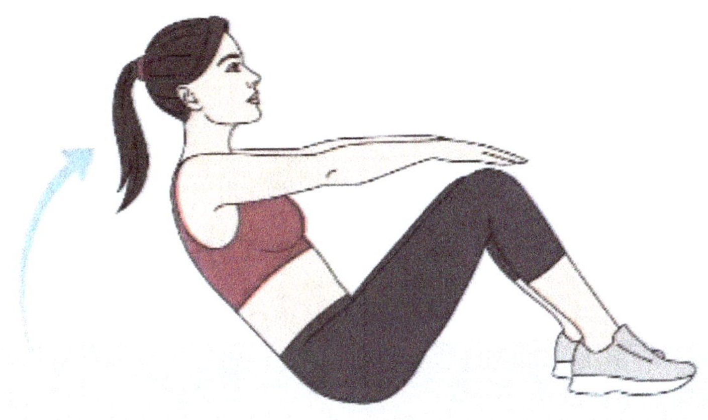

Some love this exercise, others hate it.
Lie on your back. Bend your knees and raise your legs. Tilt your pelvis so that your back lays flat on the floor without a hollow back. Put your arms behind your neck and slowly move your upper body to your knees, then put it back on the floor! With control!
Note: Do not forget to breathe!

6. PLANK
Beginner
Abdominal muscles

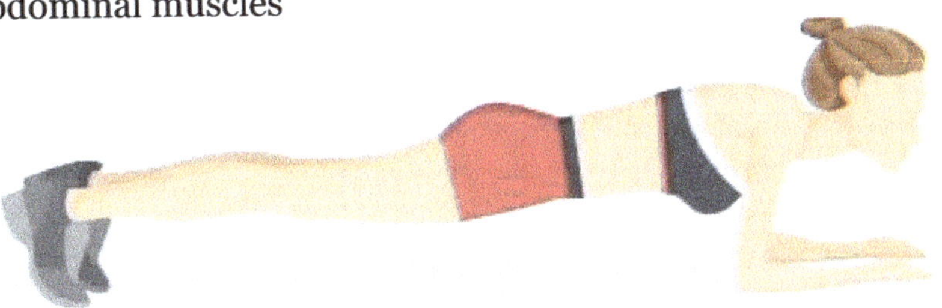

A minute has never felt so long!
Put your forearms on the floor. Lift your body so that it forms
a straight line. Hold this position. And that's it! You can try
many different variations here. For example, instead of using
your forearms, try to support yourself only wih the palms of
your hands or the side of your body!
Note: Keep your body in line! Don't sag and don't hunch your
back!

7. MOUNTAIN CLIMBER
Intermediate
Abdominal muscles

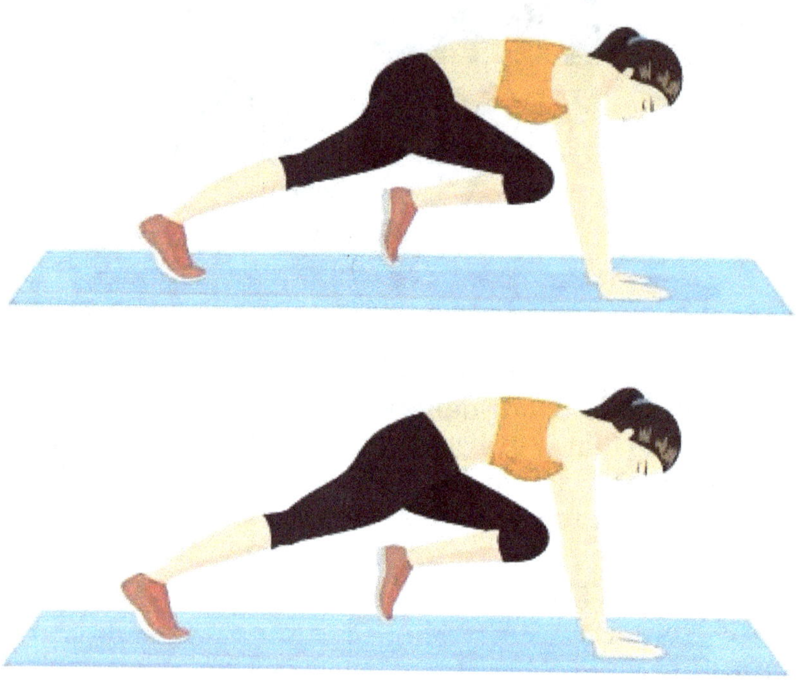

Start with a plank position (see above). Now slowly pull your
knees up to your chin, one after the other. Carry out this
movement in a controlled manner and do not stress yourself.
The slower you do this exercise, the more you will feel it in
your abs!
Note: slow, controlled movements!

8. SQUAT
Beginner

Quads, Glutes

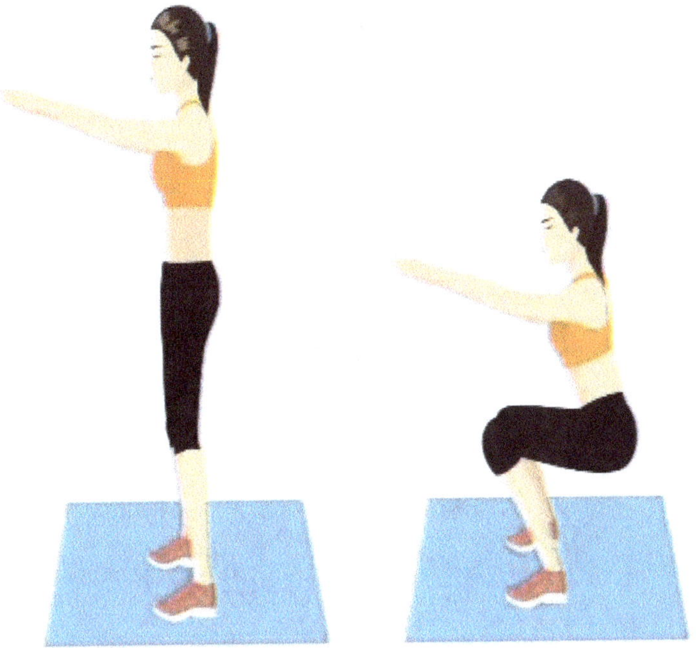

This so-called "Compound Movement" has an amazing reputation with both bodybuilders and amateur athletes! Stand on your mat a little wider than shoulder width. Crouch down and tense your buttocks when you get up!
Note: Straight back, deep squat!

9. HIP THRUST
Intermediate
Glutes

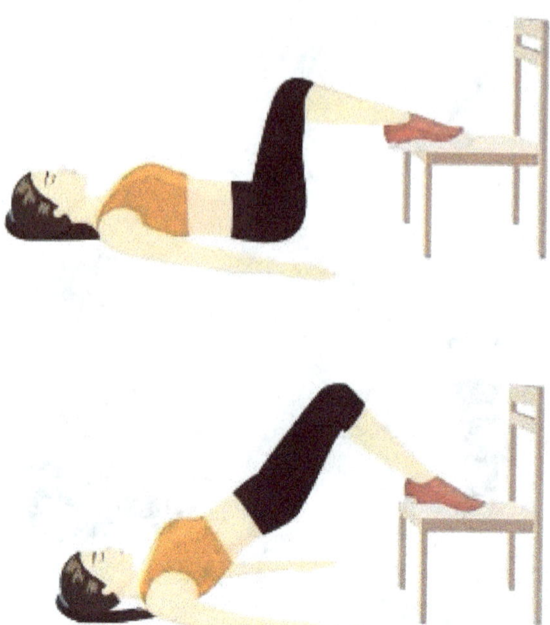

An insider tip for a firm bottom! There are two variations of this exercise.
1. Lie flat on your back, place your feet close to your butt and push your hips up.
2. Take a chair to help: place your legs on the chair and repeat the exercise as described. Due to the increased angle, this variation is a little more difficult.
Note: Adjust the position of your feet so that you feel the exercise mainly in your buttocks and not in your knees!

10. WALKING LUNGES
Intermediate
Quads

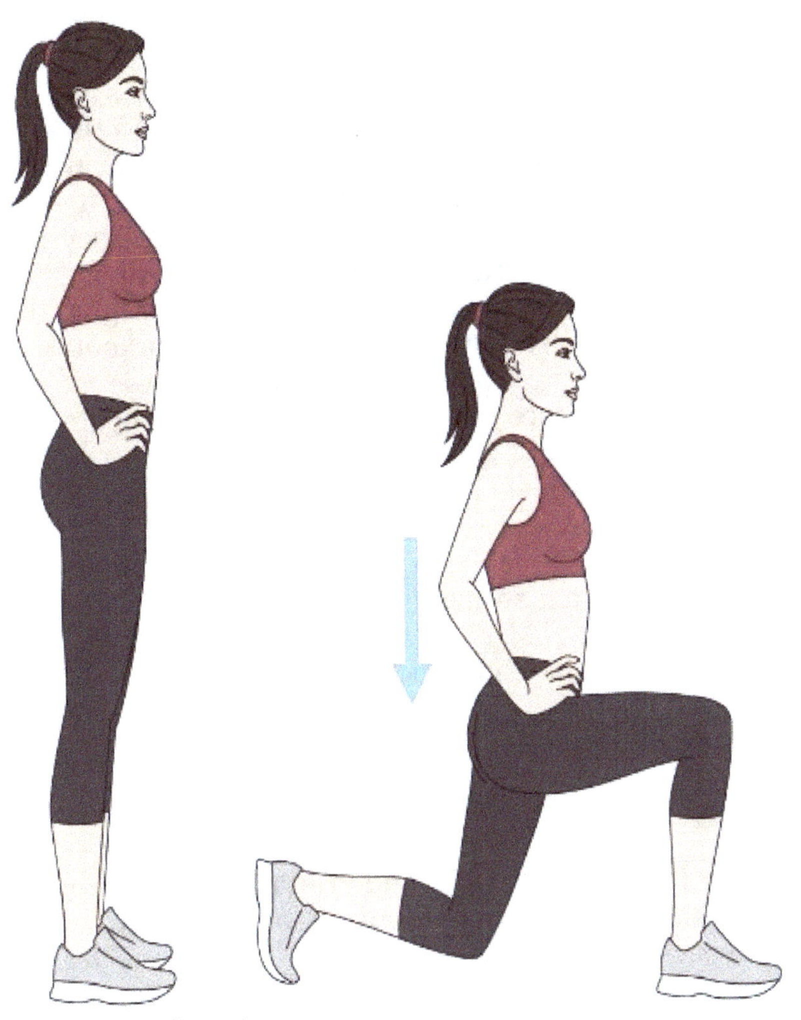

Last but not least!
If you do not feel your thighs by now, you will definitely do it after this exercise! Stand tall on your mat. Take a step forward; making sure that your knee does not protrude over the tips of your toes. Then you push yourself off with your back leg, guide it past your other leg and take another step forward. Repeat this process again and again!
Note: Never let your knees go over the tip of your toes!

5 Health-Related Components of Fitness

The five factors of fitness contribute to physical fitness and help guide the process of getting fit. You already know that benefits come when you prioritize physical activity. The trick understands what "fitness" is and how you can achieve it. That's where the five components of fitness come in. They are the blueprint for the American College of Sports Medicine (ACSM) physical activity guidelines and serve as a helpful tool for organizing and executing your well-balanced workout routine. Creating a fitness plan that incorporates these elements can help ensure you get the most health benefits from your routine.

Five Factors of Fitness

- Cardiovascular endurance

- Muscular strength

- Muscular endurance

- Flexibility

- Body composition

The Centers for Disease Control and Prevention (CDC) links regular physical activity to a reduced risk of cardiovascular disease, type 2 diabetes, some cancers, improved bone health, enhanced mental health, and improved quality of life with age. Learn more about the five components of fitness and examples.

Cardiovascular Endurance

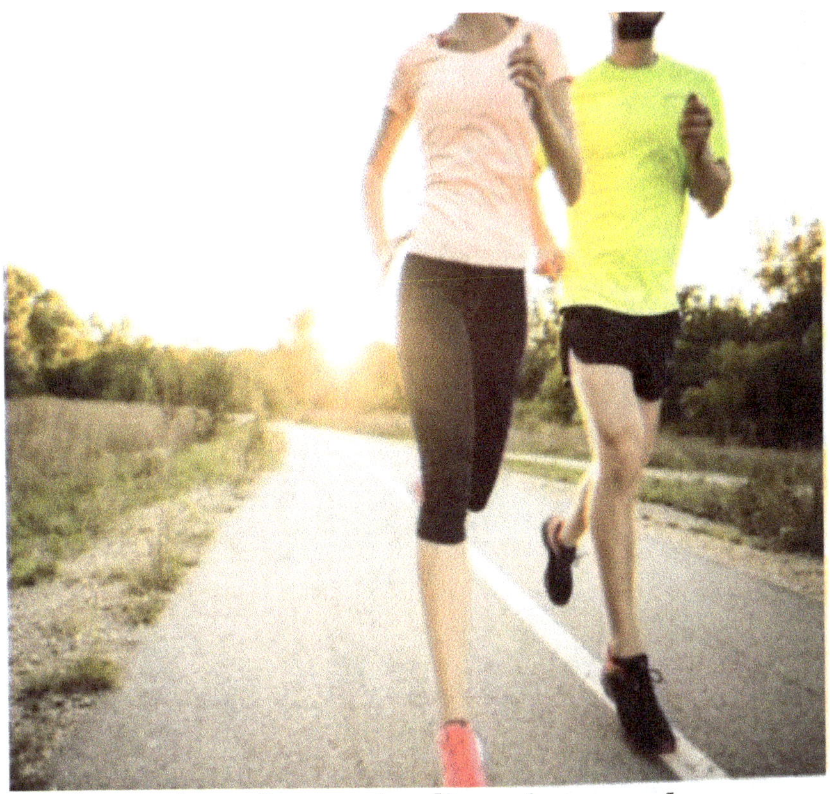

Cardiovascular endurance (cardiorespiratory endurance or aerobic fitness) refers to your body's ability to efficiently and effectively intake oxygen and deliver it to your body's tissues through the heart, lungs, arteries, vessels, and veins.3 By engaging in regular exercise that challenges your heart and lungs, you can:4

- Maintain or improve the efficient delivery and uptake of oxygen to your body's systems

- Enhance cellular metabolism

- Ease the physical challenges of everyday life

Since heart disease accounts for roughly 630,000 deaths in the United States each year, starting a workout program that enhances cardiovascular fitness is particularly important.4 Running, walking, cycling, swimming, dancing, circuit training, and boxing are a few workouts that can benefit heart health.

The key, of course, is consistency. It may sound like a lot, but 150 minutes breaks down to just 20 to 30 minutes of exercise daily, five to seven days a week.

Muscular Endurance

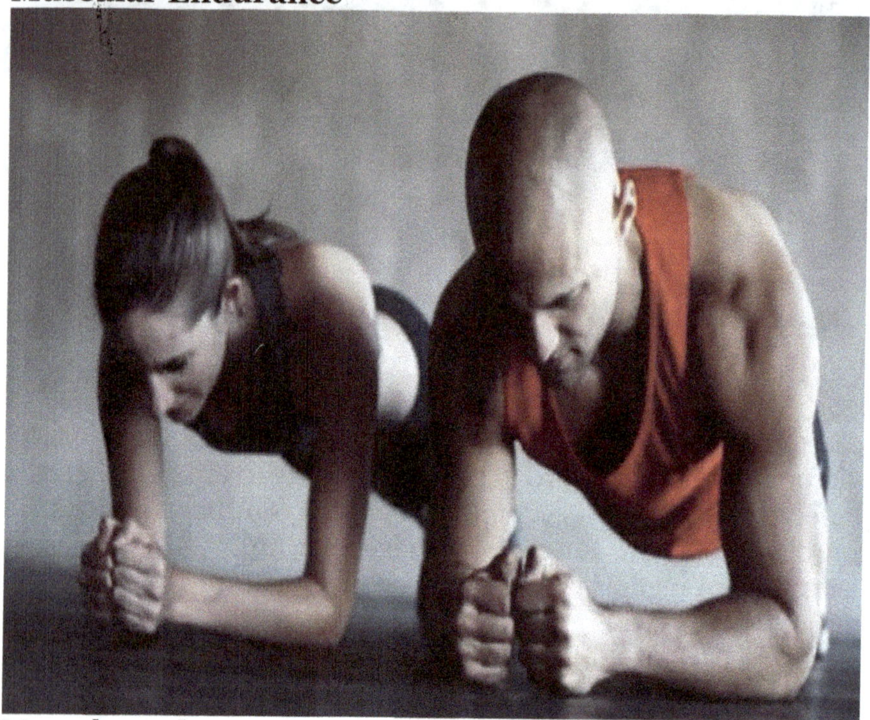

Muscular endurance is one of two factors that contribute to overall muscular health (muscular strength is the other). Think of muscular endurance as a particular muscle group's ability to continuously contract against a given resistance. Long-distance cycling offers a clear example. To pedal a bike over a long distance, often up steep inclines, cyclists must develop fatigue-resistant muscles in their legs and glutes. These are evidence of a high level of muscular endurance.

Likewise, holding a plank to develop core strength is another example of muscular endurance using isometric exercise. The longer you can contract your abdominals and keep your body in a steady position, the greater endurance you have through your hips, abs, and shoulders.

The extent to which you focus on muscular endurance should be directly related to your health or fitness goals. It's important to realize that muscular endurance is muscle group specific.

This means you can develop high endurance levels in some muscle groups (like cyclists building endurance in their legs) without necessarily acquiring the same endurance level in other muscle groups, depending on your needs.

For Everyday Health

For general health, you may want to develop enough endurance to climb up several flights of stairs or lift and carry groceries from your car to your house. Low-intensity weight-bearing or strength-training workouts will help you build up that endurance.

For Fitness-Related Goals

Suppose you want to become an endurance athlete capable of competing in sports that require continual muscle contraction, such as obstacle course races, CrossFit, or cycling. In that case, you'll need a higher level of muscular endurance. You may want to focus more on training regimens that use high-repetition strength training and sport-specific activity to make you a better athlete.

Muscular Strength

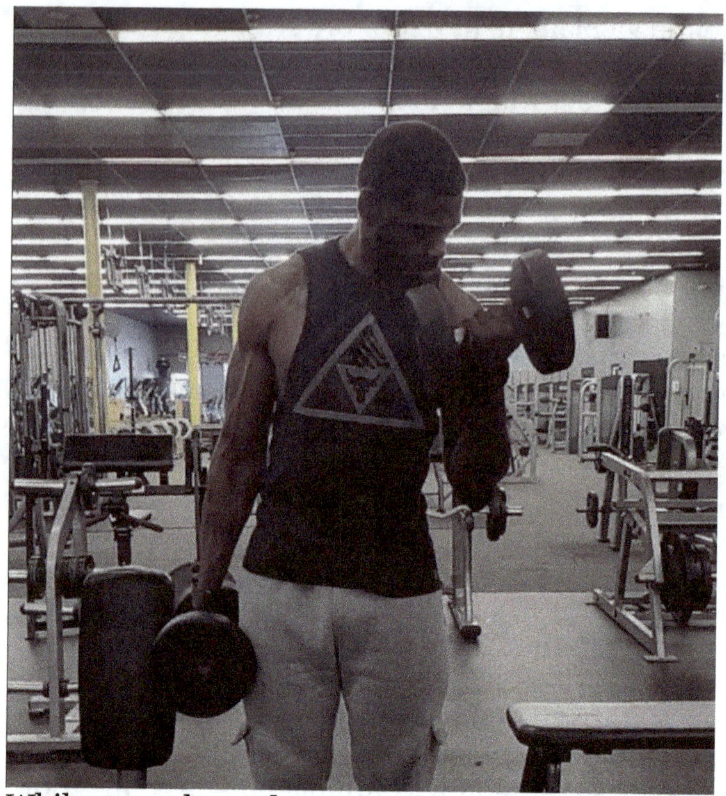

While muscular endurance refers to how fatigue-resistant a particular muscle group is, muscular strength refers to the amount of force a specific muscle group can produce in one, all-out effort. In strength training terms, it's your one-rep max.

Like muscular endurance, muscular strength is muscle group specific. In other words, you may have strong glutes but comparatively weak deltoids, or powerful pectoral muscles but comparatively weak hamstrings. This is why a well-balanced strength training program that targets all your major muscle groups is essential.

Consider Your Goals

Again, the extent to which you train for strength is determined by your health and fitness goals. For instance, if your focus is on health, you should be strong enough to lift a heavy box or easily stand up from a chair.8 In this circumstance, enhanced muscular strength may be a byproduct of a workout routine focused on developing muscular endurance.

If, however, you want to develop muscle mass or to be able to lift heavier weights at the gym, you should focus your training regimen more on lifting heavy weights.

It's possible to improve muscular strength and endurance at the same time. You can do this in conjunction with cardiovascular training. For instance, circuit-training routines that combine strength exercises and cardio into a single training bout can make your exercise program more efficient.

Flexibility

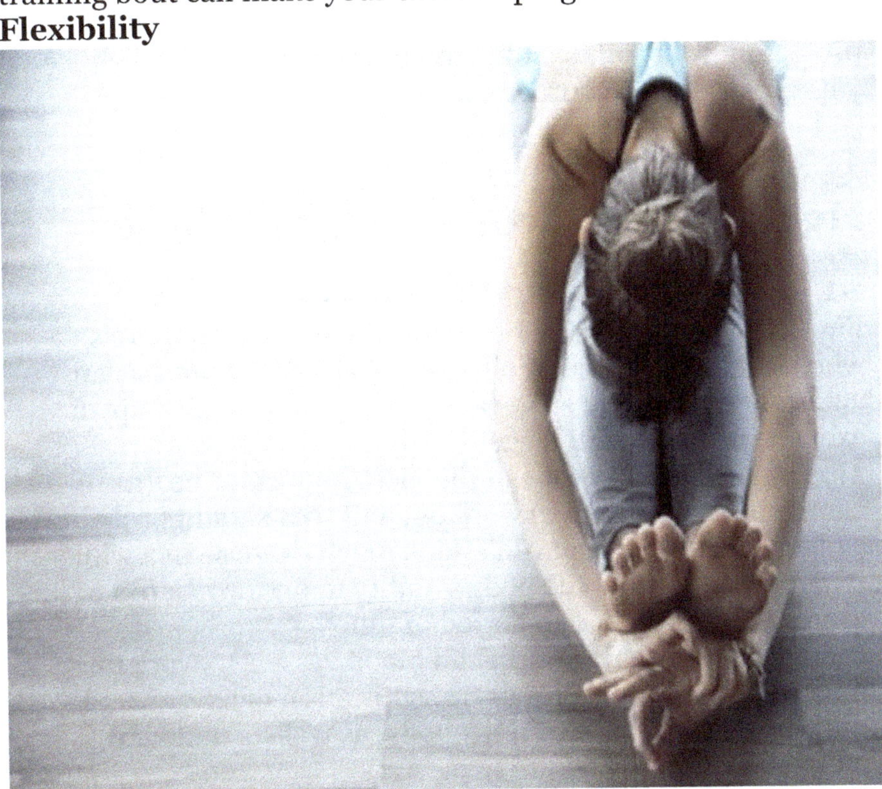

Flexibility refers to the range of motion around a given joint without pain. Like muscular strength and endurance, flexibility is joint-specific. For instance, you may have very flexible shoulders but tight and inflexible hamstrings or hips. Flexibility is essential at any age. It plays a role in unhindered movement and can affect your balance, coordination, and agility. Maintaining a full range of motion through your major joints can reduce the likelihood of injury and enhance athletic performance.

As you get older, the importance of flexibility becomes even more apparent. Think of older individuals: Many may walk with a shuffle or have difficulty reaching their arms over their heads.

This may affect the quality of life, making it more challenging to perform activities of daily living, such as reaching items on high shelves, picking up things off the floor, or simply catching their balance if they start to fall.

While completely stopping the aging process isn't possible, protecting your joints and maintaining mobility can help keep you spry well into your later years.

Health-related components of fitness

#1 - Cardiovascular Endurance

First things first, we all know how difficult it is to exercise when our lungs feel like collapsing. Lack of cardiovascular endurance is usually what causes many of us to give up on exercise when it starts to get tough...

This is what makes it one of the most important health-related components of fitness to work on, and so it should probably be a high priority if you haven't done much exercise in a while.

In simple terms, it's the body's ability to perform aerobic exercise for an extended period of time.

It relies on the heart, lungs, and blood vessels to work in unison to ensure the proper transportation of oxygen and nutrients to tissues within the body, as well as removing metabolic waste.

By strengthening the function of your cardiovascular/circulatory system through regular exercise, you can significantly improve your cardio endurance (and therefore your ability to perform long-duration or high-intensity exercise!).

How to Test Your Cardiovascular Endurance

There are a few methods that have been proven to work well for testing cardio endurance.

It's plain to see why as a fitness enthusiast or newbie, you would want to learn how to test your cardiovascular endurance; it is one of the components of fitness that people struggle with the most when beginning a new training routine. Those new to fitness will want to improve it to feel fitter and more in control of their body, while those who have been training for a while typically want to improve it to compete in intense sporting events such as a marathon or triathlon.

It's important to identify your current cardio endurance before trying to train it, as you can monitor your progress and push harder in each session.

There are a few different test methods, but one of the best to try is the Three-Minute Step test.

The Three-Minute Step test is one of the quickest ways of testing this component of fitness. To complete it, you need a 12-inch step/bench, stopwatch, and a metronome (which you can find for free online).

Method:

- Measure your pulse beforehand (1 minute)

- Set the metronome to 96 and follow the beat

- Use the bench to step up and down consistently within the time frame

- Count your pulse afterwards (1 minute)

- Measure how long it takes for your heart rate to return from this rate to normal, then record the difference

Now you know how to test your cardiovascular endurance, there's no stopping you from making the progress you want to see!

Benefits of Cardiovascular Endurance Training

As one of the most important health-related components of fitness, it's fair to say that cardio endurance has its benefits when trained regularly.

Not only can it increase your general exercise capability (therefore aiding how well the other components of fitness work), but it protects you from several health risks further down the line.

Cardio endurance training:

- Strengthens heart muscle

- Increases lung capacity

- Regulates blood pressure

- Reduces stress/enhances mood

- Lowers unhealthy cholesterol

- Aids sleep

- Prevents obesity (gives the metabolism a boost)

Fastest Ways to Improve Cardiovascular Endurance

When looking to improve your lifestyle, it's a good idea to be armed with the fastest ways to improve cardiovascular endurance.

For cardio endurance, these exercises aren't necessarily hard to guess... however, let's jump right in. Who knows, you might find something you haven't tried before!

1 - Jogging

Jogging is a great option for those looking to work on this component of fitness, especially as it can be done either outside or on a treadmill/elliptical trainer.

The most effective way to train endurance this way is to start off with a set distance and to gradually increase this distance with each session. For example, you might start with a 15-minute run, and aim to build it up to 35 minutes within a month or two.

This is a good method for increasing cardio endurance as one of the components of fitness, and you can physically see it improving each week!

2 - Cycling

While it's slightly trickier to improve cardio endurance with cycling if you're starting from scratch, it's definitely worth a try if you prefer it to jogging.

To give it a real boost, you should ride at a speed of around 10mph. Your heart rate will soar, and your breathing will quicken as your lower body muscles ache for oxygen. This is a great sign, and you should push as far as you can, just as you would on a vigorous jog.

You might start with a 15–20-minute ride and aim to build it up as you would with running duration. As long as the duration climbs with each ride, you're working on one of your most important components of fitness!

3 - Swimming

Swimming is fantastic for improving cardio endurance as it requires work from a larger range of muscles than jogging or cycling does and burns a good amount of calories.

The best way to use it to train for this type of endurance is to swim at intervals of 50, 100, then 200 yards, with short rest periods in between each set.

As with the previous exercises, be sure to increase the length of each set whilst taking shorter rest periods as time goes on, and you'll see an improvement over time!

4 - Active Sports

Any sport that requires you to get active is good for building cardio endurance, not only physically but mentally. Some people prefer sports, especially if they are extroverted, as they are sometimes bored by solitary exercises.

Sports that are good for endurance include:

- Football

- Rugby

- Hockey

- Basketball

- Surfing

- Kayaking

#2 - Muscular Endurance

The components of fitness definition for muscular endurance focus on similar ideals as cardio endurance. However, there are some differences mainly because of how unalike the cardio muscles and skeletal muscles are.

Muscular endurance refers to the fatigue resisting ability of skeletal muscles when they are contracted using less than the maximal force for an extended time period.

In other words, it measures how long a muscle is able to tolerate a high amount of repetitions with a light weight (rather than aiming for 7-12 reps with a heavy weight).

When training and learning how to test your muscular endurance, you should have a holistic approach (especially if you're into sports or looking to compete in fitness events). Endurance is different to strength, and strength is different to tone. What they all have in common though is that they complement each other when trained in unison, and you shouldn't train one without the other if you're looking for optimal results!

Muscular endurance is often the most overlooked out of the three, so it's definitely worth learning both how to test your muscular endurance and how to improve it.

How to Test Your Muscular Endurance

You may be shredded and not feel the need to test this, or you may be a newbie eager to give it a try...

No matter your skill level, you should definitely check out where you stand with one of the most important health-related components of fitness. After all, it can help you out in a number of everyday life situations as well as during exercise and sports!

One great way of learning how to test your muscular endurance is by checking out the Push-up Test.

This is a simple yet effective way of measuring the muscular endurance of most of the muscle groups in your body.

Method:

- Warm-up beforehand

- Start in a standard push-up position with your hands shoulder-width apart

- Ensure your arms are at around 90 degrees at the bottom of the push-up

- Perform as many as you can without fatiguing or breaking form

- Record your total amount of push-ups and compare them to the average amount for your gender and age!

Benefits of training muscular endurance

Muscular endurance isn't just about training your muscles to sustain long periods of training, although this is one of the most focused on benefits of training muscular endurance! When done frequently, it actually works to prevent injury, age-related decline in muscle, and a host of other things. This is what makes it one of the best health-related components of fitness to work on within our list.

1 - Push-ups

You'll notice that this is the exercise mentioned the most when you're looking at how to test your muscular endurance, so it's no surprise that it's also used to train it!

Push-ups target many muscles in your body (being a total body exercise), so they should be one of your go-to exercises when looking to train your muscles in this way...

2 - Planks

Planks will improve the endurance of your glutes, back, shoulders, hamstrings, and abs. They're similar to push-ups in this sense, but definitely serve as a great way to mix things up. You can alternate between planks and moving planks for progression, and side planks also work a treat for your obliques!

3 - Squats

Want to exercise to improve muscular endurance in your legs/lower body? If so, you can't go wrong with squats. They work your glutes, quads, hamstrings, obliques, abs, and more. Just be sure to engage your abs and glutes for the best results. You can start out with bodyweight squats, and then progress to barbell front or back squats when you're more confident!

4 - Sit-ups

Who said that muscular endurance in your core wasn't as important as the rest?...

As long as you engage your core properly and perform the correct amount of reps, you'll be able to reap the benefits and truly use this exercise to improve muscular endurance.

We'd recommend 3 sets of 10-20 reps if you're training for endurance. However, if you want to use sit-ups to build muscular strength and tone in the core, stick to around 7-10 reps at a time. Always perform 3 sets and no more than this!

5 - Lunges

Lunges are a great lower body exercise to improve muscular endurance and are arguably as effective as squats. In fact, they actually train the inner thigh muscles that are difficult to reach through other exercises.

They work your hip flexors, quads, hamstrings, glutes, and core, but only if you engage the core and glutes properly (as we keep saying!).

If you're looking to train for exercises such as running, active sports, powerlifting, etc. then this exercise will be essential for developing that lower body endurance.

#3 - Strength

When taking a good look at the health-related components of fitness, they usually confuse strength and muscular endurance. Just in case you haven't quite picked up on it yet, here's a quick recap:

Muscular endurance refers to how long your muscles can work for without fatiguing, while muscular strength is all about how much force your muscles can exert in one blow.

We're about to explain more below, so don't panic if you're scratching your head and wondering how strength training is different to training muscular endurance.

How to Test Your Muscular Strength

Testing your muscular strength is a little more complicated than testing the components of fitness that we've already covered. It relies heavily on which muscle group you want to test the strength of, so there isn't really a holistic approach! However, here are some tips to teach you how to test your muscular strength effectively:

- Select the muscles/muscle group that you wish to test the strength of

- Choose a weight or resistance that you can use multiple times before fatigue (for 7-10 reps)

- Work to exhaustion (you can't perform any more reps)

- Record how many reps you reached, and the weight used

- Use the results to estimate your 1RM (one repetition maximum)

Let's say you deadlifted 20kg for 7 reps, and then your muscles fatigued. Your 1RM equation would look something like this:
(0.033 x 7 x 20) + 20 = 24.62
24.62 is approximately 25kg, so this would be the maximum weight that you could lift for deadlifts.
You can use this equation to test pretty much any strength exercise, particularly with weights.
Your 1RM will increase with time as you train strength regularly. Now that you know how to test your muscular strength you can check on it every few weeks and increase your load!

Health Benefits of Muscular Strength Training

It's no secret that training strength has a great impact on body composition and performance in active sports.

However, if you need one final push to zone in on this area, you should check out the health benefits of muscular strength training. You may be surprised!

Strength training:

- Builds and maintains muscle mass as you age

- Boosts mood and energy levels

- Aids bone health

- Burns excess calories (improves metabolic rate)

- Shreds excess fat stores

- Improves other components of fitness (cardiovascular endurance, coordination, and balance)

Components of Fitness: Strength and How to Build It

When we talk about building strength, a quick way to approach it would be to perform similar exercises to those that build muscular endurance, but to switch the 'go for as long as you can' method to a set amount of reps at higher intensity.

If you want to progress from only bodyweight training to exercises that will take strength training further, then here's a quick-fire list to try out:

- Bicep curls with dumbbells

- Dumbbell rows

- Barbell squats

- Deadlifts

- Barbell lunges

- Pull-ups

- Triceps dips

#4 - Flexibility

This is where things start to get fun for those who want to try something different with their current routine!

You don't have to start doing backflips in the gym to work on flexibility, mind. What we mean by flexibility in this scenario is more to do with how your joints move through their full ROM (range of motion).

The main reason for flexibility being a little different to the previously mentioned components of fitness is that it's more about your body's ability to move rather than how it looks and performs and is often trained by stretching.

How to Test For Flexibility

Whether you're looking up how to test for flexibility for yourself or a client, we've got everything you need to know in this section.

The most common way to test flexibility is through the sit and reach test. It doesn't require a lot of time but can give you an accurate idea of how flexible you are, and also be used to measure your progress from flexibility training.

Tips for the sit and reach test:

- Complete the test without shoes for accurate results

- Keep your legs and knees straight, and have your feet flat against the box

- When leaning forward, do it slowly and steadily

- Be sure to reach as far as you can

- Repeat the test three times, and calculate the average result

Long Term Benefits of Flexibility Training

Sure, the long-term benefits of flexibility training could involve being able to perform all the handstands and cartwheels you thought you'd never be able to do. However, this shouldn't be your only focus!

Flexibility training has many benefits, including those that aid your health rather than giving you the ability to do party tricks. Check them out below:

- Increases athletic performance (due to growing ROM (range of motion)

- Reduces chance of injury during physical activity

- Eases muscle aches, pains, and cramps

- Improves balance and posture

Quickens recovering after exercising (improves blood flow)

Exercises to Improve Your Flexibility

Flexibility is one of the most important health-related components of fitness as it ties a lot of the more physically demanding aspects together (such as training for strength and endurance).

Flexibility exercises can be used both pre- and post-workout to stretch your connective tissues and lengthen them with regular practice. This boosts you range of motion and ability to perform other exercises.

The best exercises to improve your flexibility are as follows.

1 - Dynamic warm-ups

Dynamic warm-ups such as lunges, toe touches, bridges, hip flexor stretches, etc. are a great starting point for those looking for exercises to improve their flexibility.

They target specific muscle groups and joints over time and cause them to loosen up and move more freely.

2 - Yoga

If you're looking for a super-effective yet low-impact method of improving your flexibility, yoga should be at the top of your list. The difficulty ranger from beginner to highly advanced, so it's never too early or too late to start!

You can also practice yoga at home as all you need is a mat and some video tutorials, which you can find on YouTube or various fitness sites.

3 - Dancing

The main reason for dancing being on the list of the best exercises for increasing flexibility is that the movements involved lengthen your joints and muscle tissues with regular practice.

It's one of the quickest and easiest methods, and for some the most enjoyable (especially if you enjoy working out with others).

#5 - Body Composition

Unlike some of the other health-related components of fitness, achieving an optimal body composition is actually one of the main goals of every exercise routine. Priorities can vary but keeping an eye on excess fat stores isn't often overlooked.

So, what does the term body composition actually mean?

To be more specific, body composition refers to the amount of body fat mass that you're storing in comparison to fat-free mass, which is made up of organs, muscles, and bone etc.

It's a well-known fact that a lower body fat mass to muscle mass ratio is better for your health and will ultimately make your body appear leaner and healthier.

How to Test Your Body Composition

There are a few different ways to check on your body composition, or as it is otherwise known, your body fat percentage. It may be useful to check out our article on the different types of body fat first if you want to know more about this topic!

The Complete List of Full-Body Exercises

Benefits of Full-Body Exercises

Very few exercises can truly claim the title "full-body exercise." Plenty of exercises work multiple muscle groups, but when thinking through what to include in a full-body exercise list, movement planes should also be considered. To avoid getting lost in the weeds, let's keep it simple. Your body has three planes of movement, front to back, left to right, and top to bottom. The exercises on this list don't just engage multiple muscle groups; they also create movement across all three of those planes.

Full-body exercises have several benefits, including:

- Combining cardio and strength training into one movement. This is ideal for endurance athletes or athletes who want to see their performance improve.

- These exercises can be of higher intensity and therefore help your body burn more calories and fat in a shorter period of time.

- They can be incorporated into any training routine, whether you have the best training equipment, minimal equipment like a dumbbell set, or no equipment at all.

- A full-body workout can be performed in roughly 30-45 minutes which will save you time in the gym or working out at home.

- They are easily adjustable or customizable by lowering or raising the difficulty, which is also great for accommodating any injuries.

If you're ready to give full body exercises a shot, the list below can help challenge your body and push your training to new levels.

Benefits: Burpees are a fat burner, strength builder, and cardio exercise all wrapped into one. They are high intensity and will have you huffing and puffing after a set or two.

Plank

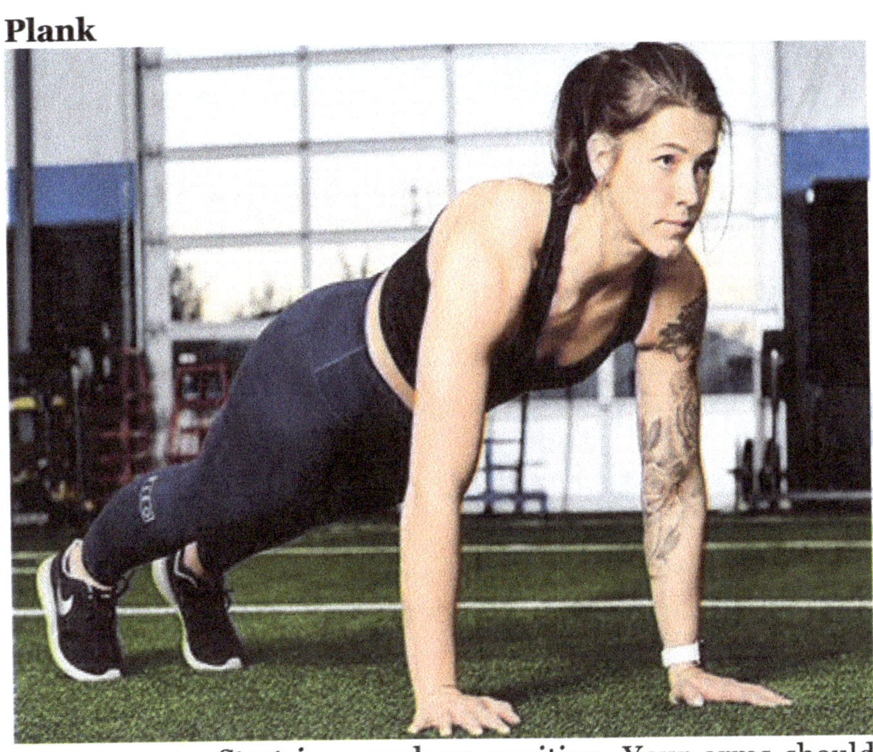

1. Start in a push-up position. Your arms should be locked out and your body a straight line from head to toe.

2. Lean forward slightly, moving your shoulders just in front of your hands. Hold this position for the allotted time, keeping your back straight and your core tight.

Benefits: Planks are one of the simplest full-body exercises, but simple does not mean easy. In a plank, you will engage almost every muscle in your body to stabilize and hold the pose. For a tougher challenge, lower yourself onto your elbows and forearms.

Hollow-Body Hold

1. Lie on your back with your legs straight and your arms extended over your head.

2. Lift your legs, arms, head, and shoulders off the ground by pressing your lower back into the ground and tightening your core.

3. Hold the pose for the allotted time, keeping your core engaged and your neck neutral.

Benefits: Hollow-body holds are primarily a core exercise, but much like the plank, you'll notice quickly that you have to tighten almost every muscle in your body to hold the pose. If you need to work up to the hollow-body hold, start with v-sits.

Hollow-Body Pull-up

1. Start with a shoulder-width overhand grip on a pull-up bar.

2. Pick up your feet and squeeze your legs together. Your legs should be fully extended in front of you like a hollow body hold.

3. Pull your chest toward the bar and pause at the top of the movement before returning to the starting position. Keep your legs extended in front of your body throughout the set.

Benefits: Pull-ups are the standard for upper-body strength since the movement requires every muscle in your upper body. However, when you add in the hollow-body hold, your core and leg muscles engage as well, making it a full-body exercise.

Handstand

1. Start in a squat position and lean forward until your hands are on the ground.

2. Slowly lift your feet off the ground until your weight is resting on your hands.

3. Maintaining your balance, slowly extend your legs until they're straight. Hold the pose.

Benefits: Like the pull-up, handstands are an upper-body dominant exercise. However, handstands also require a constantly engaged core and leg muscle chain to be performed properly. The result is a full-body exercise that will test your balance, strength, and endurance all in one movement.

Thruster

1. Start by holding a weight at your shoulders in the front rack position. Squat down, keeping the weight stabilized.

2. Press the weight overhead as you simultaneously extend your legs to rise from the squatting position.

3. Lower the weight back to the front rack position.

Benefits: Thrusters are a very versatile exercise that can be done with a dumbbell, kettlebell, barbell, or any item you can hold in two hands and feel comfortable lifting over your head. Thrusters activate muscles in all major muscle groups while also challenging your cardiovascular system, which means this exercise is a fat incinerator.

Man-Maker

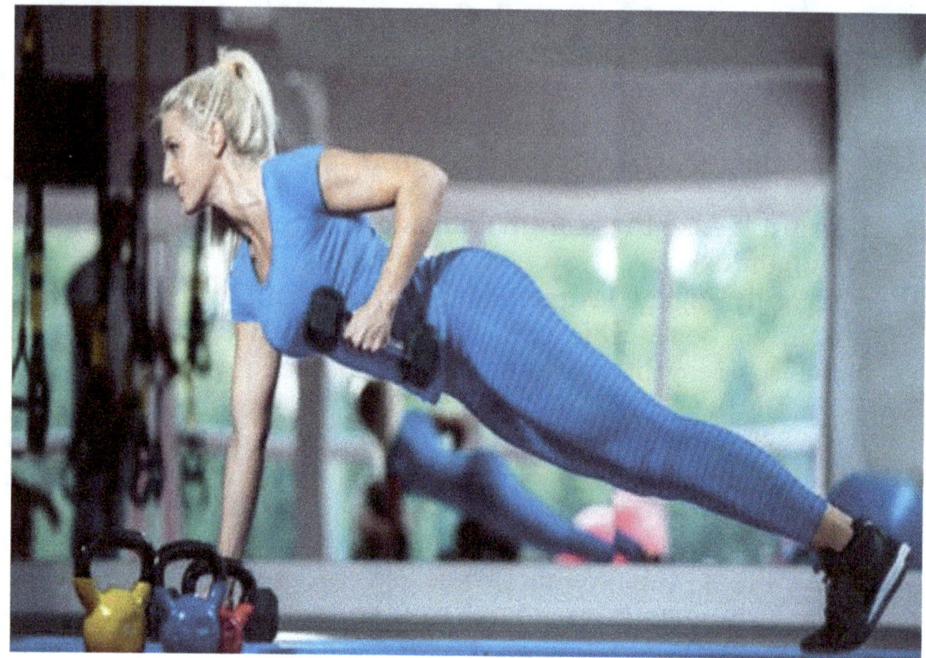

1. Start in a standing position holding a dumbbell in each hand. Set the dumbbells on the ground and kick your feet back until you're in a push-up position with your hands on the dumbbells.

2. Perform a push-up by lowering your chest to the ground and pushing back up until your arms are fully extended.

3. Perform a single-arm row with the dumbbells, one with each arm.

4. Step your feet back under your torso and lift the weights into the front rack position.

5. Press the weights overhead as you stand up from the squat position.

Benefits: Simply reading the instructions for man-makers leaves you out of breath! This movement is a combination of a burpee, a renegade row, and a thruster. In some ways it is the ultimate full-body exercise because it engages almost every muscle in your body from your toes to your shoulders.

Turkish Get-Up

1. Lie on your back with one leg bent. With the same-side hand, hold a weight over your chest with your arm straight.

2. Keeping the weight up, lift your upper body up to balance on your elbow, then straighten your arm and lift your hips off the ground so you're balancing on your hand and the side of your foot.

3. Step your other foot back and place your knee on the ground under your hips, lifting your hand off the floor so you're in a half-kneeling position.

4. With the weight still held straight overhead, straighten both legs and step your back foot forward to end in a standing position with your feet together.

5. Perform the movement in reverse to return to the starting position.

Benefits: The Turkish get-up is a difficult exercise to master, but the benefits are off the charts. You are training your legs, core, arms, shoulders, back, balance, and cardiovascular system with limited impact on your joints. Since this exercise is so complex, it's recommended that you perform it with just body weight until you get the movement down before trying it with a dumbbell or kettlebell.

Deadlift

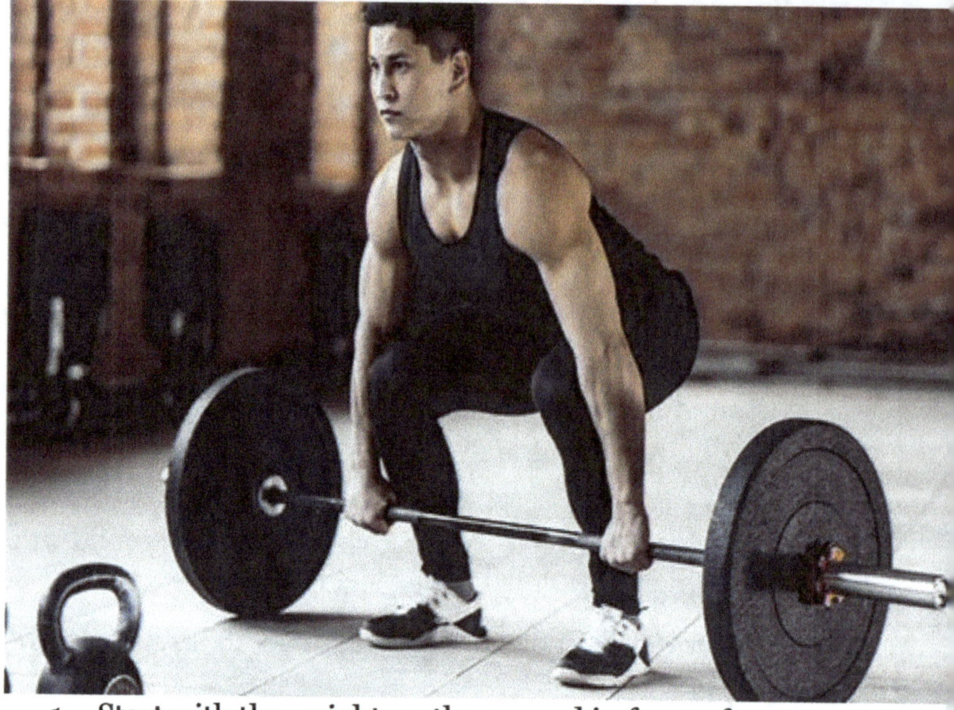

1. Start with the weight on the ground in front of you.

2. Slightly bend your knees and hinge at the hips to pick up the weight.

3. Engage your glutes as you straighten up, pulling the weight off the floor and up your shins as you return to standing. Keep your arms and back straight throughout the movement.

4. With control, lower the weight back to the floor to reset for the next rep.

Benefits: Deadlifts work through your hips, abs, and lower back, but the rest of your muscles are engaged throughout the movement, too. When done properly, deadlifts will make you feel strong and help strengthen your stabilizing muscles to improve your performance in the rest of your exercises.

Clean and Press

1. Start with the weight on the floor in front of your shins.

2. With your knees slightly bent, grip and lift the weight up your body to the front rack position in one smooth motion.

3. Press the weight overhead until your legs and arms are fully extended.

Benefits: The clean and press uses all of the major muscle groups from your feet to your shoulders to complete the movement. The first half—from floor to front rack position—targets your legs, core, and hips. The second half of the movement, the overhead press, targets your arms, chest, back, and core.

Snatch

1. Start with a barbell on the floor in front of your shins.

2. Bend your knees and hinge your hips back into a squat and grip the bar with a wide grip, almost as far as the bar will allow.

3. Keep your back flat and core tight as you stand, lifting the weight up your body in one motion from the floor to your hips.

4. When the bar reaches your hips, shrug your shoulders and drop into a squat, simultaneously bringing the barbell to an overhead position with your arms fully extended.

5. Keep the weight stabilized overhead as you straighten your legs into the standing position.

Benefits: The snatch is a dynamic exercise that requires your body's muscle groups to work together to control and balance a weight in motion. When incorporated correctly, the snatch will improve joint mobility, core stabilization, and overall strength. This is an advanced move, so try practicing it with a broom handle, PVC pipe, or empty barbell before you try it with weight. You can also try one of the snatch variations that use a dumbbell or kettle bell rather than a barbell.

Why these 10 exercises will rock your body

One surefire way to attack your fitness regimen effectively? Keep the fuss to a minimum and stick with the basics.

1. Lunges

Challenging your balance is an essential part of a well-rounded exercise routine. Lunges do just that, promoting functional movement while also increasing strength in your legs and glutes.

1. Start by standing with your feet shoulder-width apart and arms down at your sides.

2. Take a step forward with your right leg and bend your right knee as you do so, stopping when your thigh is parallel to the ground. Ensure that your right knee doesn't extend past your right foot.

3. Push up off your right foot and return to the starting position. Repeat with your left leg. This is one rep.

4. Complete 3 sets of 10 reps.

2. Pushups

1. Drop and give me 20! Pushups are one of the most basic, yet effective bodyweight moves you can perform because of the number of muscles that are recruited to perform them.

2. Start in a plank position. Your core should be tight, shoulders pulled down and back, and your neck neutral.

3. Bend your elbows and begin to lower your body down to the floor. When your chest grazes it, extend your elbows and return to the start. Focus on keeping your elbows close to your body during the movement.

4. Complete 3 sets of as many reps as possible.

If you can't quite perform a standard pushup with good form, drop down to a modified stance on your knees — you'll still reap many of the benefits from this exercise while building strength.

3. Squats

Squats increase lower body and core strength, as well as flexibility in your lower back and hips. Because they engage some of the largest muscles in the body, they also pack a major punch in terms of calories burned.

1. Start by standing straight, with your feet slightly wider than shoulder-width apart, and your arms at your sides.

2. Brace your core and, keeping your chest and chin up, push your hips back and bend your knees as if you're going to sit in a chair.

3. Ensuring your knees don't bow inward or outward, drop down until your thighs are parallel to the ground, bringing your arms out in front of you in a comfortable position. Pause for 1 second, then extend your legs and return to the starting position.

4. Complete 3 sets of 20 reps.

4. Standing overhead dumbbell presses

Compound exercises, which utilize multiple joints and muscles, are perfect for busy bees as they work several parts of your body at once. A standing overhead press isn't only one of the best exercises you can do for your shoulders, but it also engages your upper back and core.

Equipment: 10-pound dumbbells

1. Pick a light set of dumbbells — we recommend 10 pounds to start — and start by standing, either with your feet shoulder-width apart or staggered. Move the weights overhead so your upper arms are parallel to the floor.

2. Bracing your core, begin to push up until your arms are fully extended above your head. Keep your head and neck stationary.

3. After a brief pause, bend your elbows and lower the weight back down until your triceps muscle is parallel to the floor again.

4. Complete 3 sets of 12 reps.

5. Dumbbell rows

Not only will these make your back look killer in that dress, but dumbbell rows are also another compound exercise that strengthens multiple muscles in your upper body. Choose a moderate-weight dumbbell and ensure that you're squeezing at the top of the movement.

Equipment: 10-pound dumbbells

1. Start with a dumbbell in each hand. We recommend no more than 10 pounds for beginners.

2. Bend forward at the waist, so your back is at a 45-degree angle to the ground. Be certain not to arch your back. Let your arms hang straight down. Ensure your neck is in line with your back and your core is engaged.

3. Starting with your right arm, bend your elbow and pull the weight straight up toward your chest, making sure to engage your lats and stopping just below your chest.

4. Return to the starting position and repeat with the left arm. This is one rep. Repeat 10 times for 3 sets.

6. Single-leg deadlifts

This is another exercise that challenges your balance. Single-leg deadlifts require stability and leg strength. Grab a light to moderate dumbbell to complete this move.

Equipment: dumbbell

Begin standing with a dumbbell in your right hand, and your knees slightly bent.

Hinging at the hips, begin to kick your left leg straight back behind you, lowering the dumbbell down toward the ground. When you reach a comfortable height with your left leg, slowly return to the starting position in a controlled motion, squeezing your right glute. Ensure that your pelvis stays square to the ground during the movement.

Repeat 10 to 12 reps before moving the weight to your left hand and repeating the same steps on the left leg. It's suggested to do 3 sets of 10-12 reps per side.

7. Burpees

An exercise we love to hate, burpees are a super-effective, whole-body move that provides great bang for your buck for cardiovascular endurance and muscle strength.

1. Start by standing upright with your feet shoulder-width apart and your arms down at your sides.

2. With your hands out in front of you, start to squat down. When your hands reach the ground, pop your legs straight back into a pushup position.

3. Jump your feet up to your palms by hinging at the waist. Get your feet as close to your hands as you can get, landing them outside your hands if necessary.

4. Stand up straight, bringing your arms above your head, and jump.

5. This is one rep. Complete 3 sets of 10 reps as a beginner.

8. Side planks

A healthy body requires a strong core at its foundation, so don't neglect core-specific moves like the side plank.

Focus on the mind-muscle connection and controlled movements to ensure you're completing this move effectively.

1. Lie on your right side with your left leg and foot stacked on top of your right leg and foot. Prop your upper body up by placing your right forearm on the ground and elbow directly under your shoulder.

2. Contract your core to stiffen your spine and lift your hips and knees off the ground, forming a straight line with your body.

3. Return to start in a controlled manner. Repeat 3 sets of 10–15 reps on one side, then switch.

9. Planks

Planks are an effective way to target both your abdominal muscles and your whole body. Planking stabilizes your core without straining your back the way sit-ups or crunches might.

1. Begin in a pushup position with your hand and toes firmly planted on the ground, your back straight, and your core tight.

2. Keep your chin slightly tucked and your gaze just in front of your hands.

3. Take deep, controlled breaths while maintaining tension throughout your entire body, so your abs, shoulders, triceps, glutes, and quads are all engaged.

4. Complete 2-3 sets of 30-second holds to start.

10. Glute bridge

The Glute Bridge effectively works your entire posterior chain, which isn't only good for you, but it'll make your booty look perkier, too.

1. Start by lying on the floor with your knees bent, feet flat on the ground, and arms straight at your sides with your palms facing down.

2. Pushing through your heels, raise your hips off the ground by squeezing your core, glutes, and hamstrings. Your upper back and shoulders should still be in contact with the ground, and your core down to your knees should form a straight line.

3. Pause 1–2 seconds at the top and return to the starting position.

4. Complete 10–12 reps for 3 sets.

Exercise: 7 benefits of regular physical activity

Want to feel better, have more energy and even add years to your life? Just exercise.
The health benefits of regular exercise and physical activity are hard to ignore. Everyone benefits from exercise, regardless of age, sex or physical ability.
Need more convincing to get moving? Check out these seven ways that exercise can lead to a happier, healthier you.

1. Exercise controls weight
Exercise can help prevent excess weight gain or help maintain weight loss. When you engage in physical activity, you burn calories. The more intense the activity, the more calories you burn.
Regular trips to the gym are great, but don't worry if you can't find a large chunk of time to exercise every day. Any amount of activity is better than none at all. To reap the benefits of exercise, just get more active throughout your day — take the stairs instead of the elevator or rev up your household chores. Consistency is key.

2. Exercise combats health conditions and diseases

Worried about heart disease? Hoping to prevent high blood pressure? No matter what your current weight is, being active boosts high-density lipoprotein (HDL) cholesterol, the "good" cholesterol, and it decreases unhealthy triglycerides. This one-two punch keeps your blood flowing smoothly, which decreases your risk of cardiovascular diseases.

Regular exercise helps prevent or manage many health problems and concerns, including:

Stroke

Metabolic syndrome

High blood pressure

Type 2 diabetes

Depression

Anxiety

Many types of cancer

Arthritis

Falls

It can also help improve cognitive function and helps lower the risk of death from all causes.

3. Exercise improves mood

Need an emotional lift? Or need to distress after a stressful day? A gym session or brisk walk can help. Physical activity stimulates various brain chemicals that may leave you feeling happier, more relaxed and less anxious.

You may also feel better about your appearance and yourself when you exercise regularly, which can boost your confidence and improve your self-esteem.

4. Exercise boosts energy

Winded by grocery shopping or household chores? Regular physical activity can improve your muscle strength and boost your endurance.

Exercise delivers oxygen and nutrients to your tissues and helps your cardiovascular system work more efficiently. And when your heart and lung health improve, you have more energy to tackle daily chores.

5. Exercise promotes better sleep

Struggling to snooze? Regular physical activity can help you fall asleep faster, get better sleep and deepen your sleep. Just don't exercise too close to bedtime, or you may be too energized to go to sleep.

6. Exercise puts the spark back into your sex life

Do you feel too tired or too out of shape to enjoy physical intimacy? Regular physical activity can improve energy levels and increase your confidence about your physical appearance, which may boost your sex life.

But there's even more to it than that. Regular physical activity may enhance arousal for women. And men who exercise regularly are less likely to have problems with erectile dysfunction than are men who don't exercise.

7. Exercise can be fun ... and social!

Exercise and physical activity can be enjoyable. They give you a chance to unwind, enjoy the outdoors or simply engage in activities that make you happy. Physical activity can also help you connect with family or friends in a fun social setting.

So, take a dance class, hit the hiking trails or join a soccer team. Find a physical activity you enjoy, and just do it. Bored? Try something new or do something with friends or family.

Skill Related Fitness

Speed

Most sports and activities require some form of speed. Even long-distance running often requires a burst of speed to finish the race ahead of your competitors. Speed is defined as the ability to move a body part quickly. Speed is not always about how quickly you can move your whole body from A to B. It also relates to body parts. For example, when playing golf, the speed of your arms and upper body in creating the swing are vital in driving the ball over a long distance.

Reaction Time

Reaction time is how quickly your brain can respond to a stimulus and initiate a response. This is important in most sports. The most obvious being responding to the gun at the start of a race, but also a goalkeeper saving a penalty, or a badminton player reacting to a smash shot. The examples in sport are endless!

Agility

Being agile is all about being able to change your direction and the speed at which you are travelling, quickly and efficiently. This is common in sports such as football and rugby where the player with the ball dodges a defender, or in badminton or tennis, moving around the court quickly to reach the shuttlecock/ball in time.

Balance

Balance is the ability to maintain equilibrium whilst stationary or moving. Balance whilst moving is often called dynamic balance. Balance is important in all kinds of sporting situations, most notably in gymnastics and ballet but also contact sports where having good balance may prevent you from being tackled to the floor! Balance is linked to agility, as in order to quickly and efficiently change direction you must be balanced.

Coordination

Coordination is the ability to use the body parts and senses together to produce smooth efficient movements. We have all seen someone who is uncoordinated, their movement looks awkward and shaky. Being coordinated is vital in all sports, for example, hand-eye coordination in racket sports and the coordination to use the opposite arm and leg when sprinting.

Power

Power is the product of strength and speed. When we perform a task as quickly and as forcefully as we can, the result is powerful. For example, a sprint start, a shot-put or javelin throw or long-jump.

The Top 10 Benefits of Regular Exercise

Exercise is defined as any movement that makes your muscles work and requires your body to burn calories.

There are many types of physical activity, including swimming, running, jogging, walking, and dancing, to name a few.

Being active has been shown to have many health benefits, both physically and mentally. It may even help you live longer (1Trusted Source).

Here are the top 10 ways regular exercise benefits your body and brain.

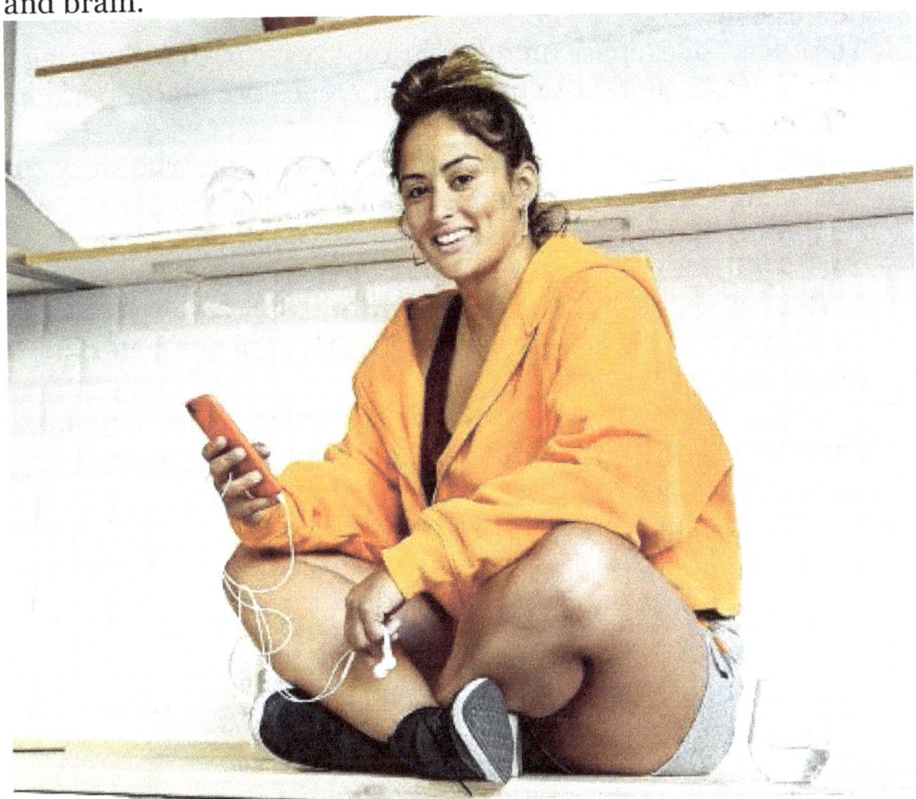

1. Exercise can make you feel happier

Exercise has been shown to improve your mood and decrease feelings of depression, anxiety, and stress.

It produces changes in the parts of the brain that regulate stress and anxiety. It can also increase brain sensitivity to the hormone's serotonin and norepinephrine, which relieve feelings of depression.

Additionally, exercise can increase the production of endorphins, which are known to help produce positive feelings and reduce the perception of pain.

Interestingly, it doesn't matter how intense your workout is. It seems that exercise can benefit your mood no matter the intensity of the physical activity.

In fact, in a study in 24 women diagnosed with depression, exercise of any intensity significantly decreased feelings of depression.

The effects of exercise on mood are so powerful that choosing to exercise (or not) even makes a difference over short periods of time.

One review of 19 studies found that active people who stopped exercising regularly experienced significant increases in symptoms of depression and anxiety, even after only a few weeks.

2. Exercise can help with weight loss

Some studies have shown that inactivity is a major factor in weight gain and obesity.

To understand the effect of exercise on weight reduction, it is important to understand the relationship between exercise and energy expenditure (spending).

Your body spends energy in three ways:

1.digesting food

2.exercising

3.maintaining body functions, like your heartbeat and breathing

While dieting, a reduced calorie intake will lower your metabolic rate, which can temporarily delay weight loss. On the contrary, regular exercise has been shown to increase your metabolic rate, which can burn more calories to help you lose weight (Trusted Source6Trusted Source, 7Trusted Source, 8Trusted Source).

Additionally, studies have shown that combining aerobic exercise with resistance training can maximize fat loss and muscle mass maintenance, which is essential for keeping the weight off and maintaining lean muscle mass.

3. Exercise is good for your muscles and bones

Exercise plays a vital role in building and maintaining strong muscles and bones.

Activities like weightlifting can stimulate muscle building when paired with adequate protein intake.

This is because exercise helps release hormones that promote your muscles' ability to absorb amino acids. This helps them grow and reduces their breakdown.

As people age, they tend to lose muscle mass and function, which can lead to an increased risk of injury. Practicing regular physical activity is essential to reducing muscle loss and maintaining strength as you age.

Exercise also helps build bone density when you're younger, in addition to helping prevent osteoporosis later in life.

Some research suggests that high impact exercise (such as gymnastics or running) or odd impact sports (such as soccer and basketball) may help promote a higher bone density than no impact sports like swimming and cycling.

4. Exercise can increase your energy levels

Exercise can be a real energy booster for many people, including those with various medical conditions.

One older study found that 6 weeks of regular exercise reduced feelings of fatigue for 36 people who had reported persistent fatigue.

And let's not forget the fantastic heart and lung health benefits of exercise. Aerobic exercise boosts the cardiovascular system and improves lung health, which can significantly help with energy levels.

As you move more, your heart pumps more blood, delivering more oxygen to your working muscles. With regular exercise, your heart becomes more efficient and adept at moving oxygen into your blood, making your muscles more efficient.

Over time, this aerobic training results in less demand on your lungs, and it requires less energy to perform the same activities — one of the reasons you're less likely to get short of breath during vigorous activity.

Additionally, exercise has been shown to increase energy levels in people with other conditions, such as cancer.

5. Exercise can reduce your risk of chronic disease

Lack of regular physical activity is a primary cause of chronic disease.

Regular exercise has been shown to improve insulin sensitivity, heart health, and body composition. It can also decrease blood pressure and cholesterol levels.

More specifically, exercise can help reduce or prevent the following chronic health conditions.

Type 2 diabetes. Regular aerobic exercise may delay or prevent type 2 diabetes. It also has considerable health benefits for people with type 1 diabetes. Resistance training for type 2 diabetes includes improvements in fat mass, blood pressure, lean body mass, insulin resistance, and glycemic control.

Heart disease. Exercise reduces cardiovascular risk factors and is also a therapeutic treatment for people with cardiovascular disease.

Many types of cancer. Exercise can help reduce the risk of several cancers, including breast, colorectal, endometrial, gallbladder, kidney, lung, liver, ovarian, pancreatic, prostate, thyroid, gastric, and esophageal cancer.

High cholesterol. Regular moderate intensity physical activity can increase HDL (good) cholesterol while maintaining or offsetting increases in LDL (bad) cholesterol. Research supports the theory that high intensity aerobic activity is needed to lower LDL levels.

Hypertension: Participating in regular aerobic exercise can lower resting systolic BP 5–7 mmHG among people with hypertension.

In contrast, a lack of regular exercise — even in the short term — can lead to significant increases in belly fat, which may increase the risk of type 2 diabetes and heart disease.

That's why regular physical activity is recommended to reduce belly fat and decrease the risk of developing these conditions.

6. Exercise can help skin health

Your skin can be affected by the amount of oxidative stress in your body.

Oxidative stress occurs when the body's antioxidant defenses cannot completely repair the cell damage caused by compounds known as free radicals. This can damage the structure of the cells and negatively impact your skin.

Even though intense and exhaustive physical activity can contribute to oxidative damage, regular moderate exercise can actually increase your body's production of natural antioxidants, which help protect cells.

In the same way, exercise can stimulate blood flow and induce skin cell adaptations that can help delay the appearance of skin aging.

7. Exercise can help your brain health and memory

Exercise can improve brain function and protect memory and thinking skills.

To begin with, it increases your heart rate, which promotes the flow of blood and oxygen to your brain. It can also stimulate the production of hormones that enhance the growth of brain cells.

Plus, the ability of exercise to prevent chronic disease can translate into benefits for your brain, since its function can be affected by these conditions.

Regular physical activity is especially important in older adults since aging — combined with oxidative stress and inflammation — promotes changes in brain structure and function.

Exercise has been shown to cause the hippocampus, a part of the brain that's vital for memory and learning, to grow in size, which may help improve mental function in older adults.

Lastly, exercise has been shown to reduce changes in the brain that can contribute to conditions like Alzheimer's disease and dementia

8. Exercise can help with relaxation and sleep quality

Regular exercise can help you relax and sleep better.

With regard to sleep quality, the energy depletion (loss) that occurs during exercise stimulates restorative processes during sleep.

Moreover, the increase in body temperature that occurs during exercise is thought to improve sleep quality by helping body temperature drop during sleep.

Many studies on the effects of exercise on sleep have reached similar conclusions.

One review of six studies found that participating in an exercise training program helped improve self-reported sleep quality and reduced sleep latency, which is the amount of time it takes to fall asleep.

One study conducted over 4 months found that both stretching, and resistance exercise led to improvements in sleep for people with chronic insomnia.

Getting back to sleep after waking, sleep duration, and sleep quality improved after both stretching and resistance exercise. Anxiety was also reduced in the stretching group.

What's more, engaging in regular exercise seems to benefit older adults, who are often affected by sleep disorders.

You can be flexible with the kind of exercise you choose. It appears that either aerobic exercise alone or aerobic exercise combined with resistance training can both improve sleep quality.

9. Exercise can reduce pain

Although chronic pain can be debilitating, exercise can actually help reduce it.

In fact, for many years, the recommendation for treating chronic pain was rest and inactivity. However, recent studies show that exercise helps relieve chronic pain.

In fact, one review of several studies found that exercise can help those with chronic pain reduce their pain and improve their quality of life.

Several studies also show that exercise can help control pain associated with various health conditions, including chronic low back pain, fibromyalgia, and chronic soft tissue shoulder disorder, to name a few.

Additionally, physical activity can also raise pain tolerance and decrease pain perception.

10. Exercise can promote a better sex life

Exercise has been proven to boost sex drive.

Engaging in regular exercise can strengthen the heart, improve blood circulation, tone muscles, and enhance flexibility, all of which can improve your sex life.

Physical activity can also improve sexual performance and sexual pleasure while increasing the frequency of sexual activity.

Interestingly enough, one study showed that regular exercise was associated with increased sexual function and desire in 405 postmenopausal women.

A review of 10 studies also found that exercising for at least 160 minutes per week over a 6-month period could help significantly improve erectile function in men.

What's more, another study found that a simple routine of a 6-minute walk around the house helped 41 men reduce their erectile dysfunction symptoms by 71%.

Yet another study demonstrated that women with polycystic ovary syndrome, which can reduce sex drive, increased their sex drive with regular resistance training for 16 weeks

Unexpected Benefits of Exercise

1. Reduce stress

Rough day at the office? Spilled coffee and got your tie stuck in the shredder? Lacey in Accounts threw stuff at you again? Chill out by taking a walk or heading to the gym for a quick workout.

One of the most common mental benefits of exercise is stress relief. Working up a sweat can help you manage physical and mental stress. Exercise also increases concentrations of norepinephrine, a chemical that can moderate your brain's response to stress.

So go ahead and get sweaty — it can reduce stress and boost your body's ability to deal with existing mental tension. Win-win! And boo to Lacey — we got your back in the Accounts beef.

2. Boost happy chemicals

Slogging through a few miles on the 'mill can be tough, but it's worth the effort.

Exercise causes your body to produce endorphins, which trigger feelings of happiness and euphoria. Research has shown that in people with major depression, exercise can increase the chance of remission by 22 percent by circulating endorphins.

For this reason, docs recommend that people dealing with depression or anxiety (or those who are just feeling blue) pencil in some gym time. A 2013 study found no difference between the effectiveness of antidepressants and exercise. Don't worry if you're not exactly the gym-rat type — working out for just 30 minutes a few times a week can instantly boost your overall mood.

3. Improve self-confidence

If you're not quite at Fonz-level self-confidence just yet, don't worry — not all of us have to jump the shark to feel great. Hopping on the treadmill can help you feel like a million bucks too.

On a very basic level, physical fitness can boost self-esteem and improve positive self-image. Regardless of weight, size, gender, or age, exercise can quickly elevate a person's perception of their attractiveness.

Exercise is your way of reminding yourself how beautiful you are. So, step on the Cross Fit and send your soul some flirty DMs!

4. Enjoy the great outdoors

For an extra boost of self-love, take your workout to the great outdoors. Exercising outside can increase self-esteem even more.

Find an outdoor workout that fits your style, whether it's rock climbing, hiking, canoeing, or just taking a jog in the park. Even a long walk-through verdant pastures and beautiful landscapes can be nourishing for your body and mind.

Plus, all that vitamin D from soaking up the sun (while wearing sunscreen, of course!) can reduce your risk of experiencing symptoms of depression.

Why book a spa day when a little fresh air and sunshine (and exercise) can work wonders for self-confidence and happiness?

5. Prevent cognitive decline

It's unpleasant, but it's true: As we get older, our brains get a little… hazy. As aging and degenerative conditions like Alzheimer's disease kill off brain cells, the noggin shrinks, damaging many important brain functions in the process.

While exercise and a healthy diet can't "cure" Alzheimer's, they can help shore up your brain against cognitive decline that begins after age 45.

Working out also boosts the chemicals that support and prevent degeneration of the hippocampus, an important part of your brain for memory and learning.

Going for a run now might help you do better in that game of bridge in 40 years.

6. Alleviate anxiety

Pop quiz, hotshot: Which is better at relieving anxiety — a warm bubble bath or a 20-minute jog?

You might be surprised at the answer. (Don't try jogging in the bath — it is not a safe pastime.)

The warm and fuzzy chemicals that start to swim around your body after exercise can help soothe people with anxiety disorders.

Hopping on the track or treadmill for some moderate-to-high intensity aerobic exercise (intervals, anyone?) can reduce anxiety symptoms. In a small 2018 study of people with a diagnosis of panic disorder, regular moderate-to-hard exercise led to a greater reduction in anxiety than light exercise.

7. Boost brainpower

Brawn and brains are not mutually exclusive. Studies have shown that cardiovascular exercise can create new brain cells and improve overall brain performance. Trusted Source (Why do you think The Hulk is so good at science?)

Ready to apply for a Nobel Prize? A 2019 study suggests that a tough workout increases levels of a brain-derived protein called BDNF, which may help with decision making, higher thinking, and learning.

8. Sharpen memory

Get ready to win big at Go Fish and Pairs: Regular physical activity boosts memory and the ability to learn new things. Working up a sweat increases production of cells in the hippocampus that are responsible for memory and learning. For this reason, research has linked children's brain development with their level of physical fitness (take that, recess haters!). Trusted Source But exercise-based brainpower isn't just for kids.

Even if it's not as fun as a game of Tag, working out can boost memory among grown-ups too. A 2006 study found that running sprints improved vocabulary retention among healthy adults. And a 2018 study found that adults performed better on memory tests after short periods of light exercise.

9. Help manage addiction

The brain releases dopamine, the "reward chemical," in response to any form of pleasure. And yes, our good friend exercise can kick off a considerable wave of dopamine. However, so do drugs and alcohol. This reward cycle in the brain can lead to patterns of substance use disorder.

Exercise is there for people while they recover from addiction. Physical activity can distract people from cravings when they're trying to quit smoking.

Working out while on the wagon has other benefits too. Excessive alcohol use disrupts many body processes, including circadian rhythms. As a result, people with alcohol use disorder may find they have trouble falling asleep without drinking.

A 2010 study on animals suggested that exercise might help reset the body clock so people can hit the hay at the right time without alcohol.

10. Get more done

Feeling uninspired in the cubicle? The solution might be just a short walk or jog away. Research suggests that workers who take time for regular exercise are more productive and have more energy than their more sedentary peers.

While busy schedules can make it tough to squeeze in a gym session in the middle of the day, some experts believe that midday is the ideal time for a workout due to the body's circadian rhythms.

What is nutrition, and why does it matter?

Nutrition

Nutrition is a critical part of health and development. Better nutrition is related to improved infant, child and maternal health, stronger immune systems, safer pregnancy and childbirth, lower risk of non-communicable diseases (such as diabetes and cardiovascular disease), and longevity.

Healthy children learn better. People with adequate nutrition are more productive and can create opportunities to gradually break the cycles of poverty and hunger.

Malnutrition, in every form, presents significant threats to human health. Today the world faces a double burden of malnutrition that includes both undernutrition and overweight, especially in low- and middle-income countries.

WHO is providing scientific advice and decision-making tools that can help countries take action to address all forms of malnutrition to support health and wellbeing for all, at all ages.

This fact file explores the risks posed by all forms of malnutrition, starting from the earliest stages of development, and the responses that the health system can give directly and through its influence on other sectors, particularly the food system.

Macronutrients

Macronutrients are nutrients that people need in relatively large quantities.

Carbohydrates

Sugar, starch, and fiber are types of carbohydrates.

Sugars are simple carbs. The body quickly breaks down and absorbs sugars and processed starch. They can provide rapid energy, but they do not leave a person feeling full. They can also cause a spike in blood sugar levels. Frequent sugar spikes increase the risk of type 2 diabetes and its complications.

Fiber is also a carbohydrate. The body breaks down some types of fiber and uses them for energy; others are metabolized by gut bacteria, while other types pass through the body.

Fiber and unprocessed starch are complex carbs. It takes the body some time to break down and absorb complex carbs. After eating fiber, a person will feel full for longer. Fiber may also reduce the risk of diabetes, cardiovascular disease, and colorectal cancer. Complex carbs are a more healthful choice than sugars and refined carbs.

Proteins

Proteins consist of amino acids, which are organic compounds that occur naturally.

There are 20 amino acids. Some of these are essential which means people need to obtain them from food. The body can make the others.

Some foods provide complete protein, which means they contain all the essential amino acids the body needs. Other foods contain various combinations of amino acids.

Most plant-based foods do not contain complete protein, so a person who follows a vegan diet needs to eat a range of foods throughout the day that provides the essential amino acids.

Fats

Fats are essential for:

- lubricating joints

- helping organs produce hormones

- enabling the body to absorb certain vitamins

- reducing inflammation

- preserving brain health

Too much fat can lead to obesity, high cholesterol, liver disease, and other health problems.

However, the type of fat a person eats makes a difference. Unsaturated fats, such as olive oil, are more healthful than saturated fats, which tend to come from animals.

Water

The adult human body is up to 60% water, and it needs water for many processes. Water contains no calories, and it does not provide energy.

Many people recommend consuming 2 liters, or 8 glasses, of water a day, but it can also come from dietary sources, such as fruit and vegetables. Adequate hydration will result in pale yellow urine.

Requirements will also depend on an individual's body size and age, environmental factors, activity levels, health status, and so on.

Click here to find out how much water a person needs each day and here to learn about the benefits of drinking water.

Micronutrients

Micronutrients are essential in small amounts. They include vitamins and minerals. Manufacturers sometimes add these to foods. Examples include fortified cereals and rice.

Minerals

The body needs carbon, hydrogen, oxygen, and nitrogen.

It also needs dietary minerals, such as iron, potassium, and so on.

In most cases, a varied and balanced diet will provide the minerals a person needs. If a deficiency occurs, a doctor may recommend supplements.

Here are some of the minerals the body needs to function well.

Potassium

Potassium is an electrolyte. It enables the kidneys, the heart, the muscles, and the nerves to work properly. The 2015–2020 Dietary Guidelines for Americans recommend that adults consume 4,700 milligrams (mg) of potassium each day.

Too little can lead to high blood pressure, stroke, and kidney stones.

Too much may be harmful to people with kidney disease.
Avocados, coconut water, bananas, dried fruit, squash, beans,
and lentils are good sources.

Sodium

Sodium is an electrolyte that helps:

- maintain nerve and muscle function

- regulate fluid levels in the body

Too little can lead to hypernatremia. Symptoms include
lethargy, confusion, and fatigue. Learn more here.
Too much can lead to high blood pressure, which increases the
risk of cardiovascular disease and stroke.
Table salt, which is made up of sodium and chloride, is a
popular condiment. However, most people consume too much
sodium, as it already occurs naturally in most foods.
Experts urge people not to add table salt to their diet. Current
guidelines recommend consuming no more than 2,300 mg of
sodium a day, or around one teaspoon.
This recommendation includes both naturally occurring
sources, as well as salt a person adds to their food. People with
high blood pressure or kidney disease should eat less.

Calcium

The body needs calcium to form bones and teeth. It also
supports the nervous system, cardiovascular health, and other
functions.
Too little can cause bones and teeth to weaken. Symptoms of a
severe deficiency include tingling in the fingers and changes in
heart rhythm, which can be life-threatening.
Too much can lead to constipation, kidney stones, and reduced
absorption of other minerals.
Current guidelines for adults recommend consuming 1,000
mg a day, and 1,200 mg for women aged 51 and over.
Good sources include dairy products, tofu, legumes, and
green, leafy vegetables

Phosphorus

Phosphorus is present in all body cells and contributes to the
health of the bones and teeth.

Too little phosphorus can lead to bone diseases, affect appetite, muscle strength, and coordination. It can also result in anemia, a higher risk of infection, burning or prickling sensations in the skin, and confusion.

Too much in the diet is unlikely to cause health problems though toxicity is possible from supplements, medications, and phosphorus metabolism problems.

Adults should aim to consume around 700 mg of phosphorus each day. Good sources include dairy products, salmon, lentils, and cashews.

Magnesium

Magnesium contributes to muscle and nerve function. It helps regulate blood pressure and blood sugar levels, and it enables the body to produce proteins, bone, and DNA.

Too little magnesium can eventually lead to weakness, nausea, tiredness, restless legs, sleep conditions, and other symptoms.

Too much can result in digestive and, eventually, heart problems.

Nuts, spinach, and beans are good sources of magnesium. Adult females need 320 mg of magnesium each day, and adult males need 420 mg.

Zinc

Zinc plays a role in the health of body cells, the immune system, wound healing, and the creation of proteins.

Too little can lead to hair loss, skin sores, changes in taste or smell, and diarrhea, but this is rare.

Too much can lead to digestive problems and headaches. Click here to learn more.

Adult females need 8 mg of zinc a day, and adult males need 11 mg. Dietary sources include oysters, beef, fortified breakfast cereals, and baked beans. For more on dietary sources of zinc, click here.

Iron

Iron is crucial for the formation of red blood cells, which carry oxygen to all parts of the body. It also plays a role in forming connective tissue and creating hormones.

Too little can result in anemia, including digestive issues, weakness, and difficulty thinking. Learn more here about iron deficiency.

Too much can lead to digestive problems, and very high levels can be fatal.

Good sources include fortified cereals, beef liver, lentils, spinach, and tofu. Adults need 8 mg of iron a day, but females need 18 mg during their reproductive years.

Manganese

The body uses manganese to produce energy it plays a role in blood clotting, and it supports the immune system.

Too little can result in weak bones in children, skin rashes in men, and mood changes in women.

Too much can lead to tremors, muscle spasms, and other symptoms, but only with very high amounts.

Mussels, hazelnuts, brown rice, chickpeas, and spinach all provide manganese. Male adults need 2.3 mg of manganese each day, and females need 1.8 mg.

Copper

Copper helps the body makes energy and produces connective tissues and blood vessels.

Too little copper can lead to tiredness, patches of light skin, high cholesterol, and connective tissue disorders. This is rare.

Too much copper can result in liver damage, abdominal pain, nausea, and diarrhea. Too much copper also reduces the absorption of zinc.

Good sources include beef liver, oysters, potatoes, mushrooms, sesame seeds, and sunflower seeds. Adults need 900 micrograms (mcg) of copper each day.

Selenium

Selenium is made up of over 24 selenoproteins, and it plays a crucial role in reproductive and thyroid health. As an antioxidant, it can also prevent cell damage.

Too much selenium can cause garlic breath, diarrhea, irritability, skin rashes, brittle hair or nails, and other symptoms.

Too little can result in heart disease, infertility in men, and arthritis.

Adults need 55 mcg of selenium a day.

Brazil nuts are an excellent source of selenium. Other plant sources include spinach, oatmeal, and baked beans. Tuna, ham, and enriched macaroni are all excellent sources.

Vitamins

People need small amounts of various vitamins. Some of these, such as vitamin C, are also antioxidants. This means they help protect cells from damage by removing toxic molecules, known as free radicals, from the body.

Vitamins can be:

Water-soluble: The eight B vitamins and vitamin C

Fat-soluble: Vitamins A, D, E, and K

Water soluble vitamins

People need to consume water-soluble vitamins regularly because the body removes them more quickly, and it cannot store them easily.

Vitamin	Effect of too little	Effect of too much	Sources
B-1 (thiamin)	Beriberi Wernicke-Korsakoff syndrome	Unclear, as the body excretes it in the urine.	Fortified cereals and rice, pork, trout, black beans
B-2 (riboflavin)	Hormonal problems, skin disorders, swelling in the mouth and throat	Unclear, as the body excretes it in the urine.	Beef liver, breakfast cereal, oats, yogurt, mushrooms, almonds
B-3 (niacin)	Pellagra, including skin changes, red tongue, digestive and neurological symptoms	Facial flushing, burning, itching, headaches, rashes, and dizziness	Beef liver, chicken breast, brown rice, fortified cereals, peanuts.
B-5 (pantothenic acid)	Numbness and burning in hands and feet, fatigue, stomach pain	Digestive problems at high doses.	Breakfast cereal, beef liver, shiitake mushroom, sunflower seeds
B-6 (pyridoxamine, pyridoxal)	Anemia, itchy rash, skin changes, swollen tongue	Nerve damage, loss of muscle control	Chickpeas, beef liver, tuna, chicken breast, fortified cereals, potatoes

Vitamin	Effect of too little	Effect of too much	Sources
B-7 (biotin)	Hair loss, rashes around the eyes and other body openings, conjunctivitis	Unclear	Beef liver, egg, salmon, sunflower seeds, sweet potato
B-9 (folic acid, folate)	Weakness, fatigue, difficulty focusing, heart palpitations, shortness of breath	May increase cancer risk	Beef liver, spinach, black-eyed peas, fortified cerea asparagus
B-12 (cobalamins)	Anemia, fatigue, constipation, weight loss, neurological changes	No adverse effects reported	Clams, beef liver, fortified yeasts, plant milks, and breakfast cereals, some o fish.
Vitamin C (ascorbic acid)	Scurvy, including fatigue, skin rash, gum inflammation, poor wound healing	Nausea, diarrhea, stomach cramps	Citrus fruits, berries, red a green peppers, kiwi fruit, broccoli, baked potatoes, fortified juices.

Fat-soluble vitamins

The body absorbs fat-soluble vitamins through the intestines with the help of fats (lipids). The body can store them and does not remove them quickly. People who follow a low-fat diet may not be able to absorb enough of these vitamins. If too many build up, problems can arise.

Vitamin	Effect of too little	Effect of too much	Sources
Vitamin A (retinoids)	Night blindness	Pressure on the brain, nausea, dizziness, skin irritation, joint and bone pain, orange pigmented skin color	Sweet potato, beef liver, spinach, and other dark leafy greens, carrots, wir squash
Vitamin D	Poor bone formation and weak bones	Anorexia, weight loss, changes in heart rhythm, damage to cardiovascular system and kidneys	Sunlight exposure plus dietary sources: cod live oil, oily fish, dairy produc fortified juices
Vitamin E	Peripheral neuropathy, retinopathy, reduced immune response	May reduce the ability of blood to clot	Wheatgerm, nuts, seeds, sunflower and safflower spinach
Vitamin K	Bleeding and hemorrhaging in severe cases	No adverse effects but it may interact with blood thinners and other drugs	Leafy, green vegetables, soybeans, edamame, okr natto

Multivitamins are available for purchase in stores or online, but people should speak to their doctor before taking any supplements, to check that they are suitable for them to use.

Antioxidants

Some nutrients also act as antioxidants. These may be vitamins, minerals, proteins, or other types of molecules. They help the body remove toxic substances known as free radicals, or reactive oxygen species. If too many of these substances remain in the body, cell damage and disease can result.

Dietitian vs. nutritionist

A registered dietitian nutritionist (RD or RDN) studies food, nutrition, and dietetics. To become a registered dietitian, a person needs to attend an accredited university, follow an approved curriculum, complete a rigorous internship, pass a licensure exam, and complete 75 or more continuing education hours every 5 years. Dietitians work in private and public healthcare, education, corporate wellness, research, and the food industry.

A nutritionist learns about nutrition through self-study or formal education, but they do not meet the requirements to use the titles RD or RDN. Nutritionists often work in the food industry and in food science and technology.

Health and Nutrition Tips That Are Actually Evidence-Based

It's easy to get confused when it comes to health and nutrition. Even qualified experts often seem to hold opposing opinions, which can make it difficult to figure out what you should actually be doing to optimize your health.

1. Limit sugary drinks

Sugary drinks like sodas, fruit juices, and sweetened teas are the primary source of added sugar in the American diet. Unfortunately, findings from several studies point to sugar-sweetened beverages increasing risk of heart disease and type 2 diabetes, even in people who are not carrying excess body fat.

Sugar-sweetened beverages are also uniquely harmful for children, as they can contribute not only to obesity in children but also to conditions that usually do not develop until adulthood, like type 2 diabetes, high blood pressure, and non-alcoholic fatty liver disease.

Healthier alternatives include:

Water

Unsweetened teas

Sparkling water

Coffee

2. Eat nuts and seeds

Some people avoid nuts because they are high in fat. However, nuts and seeds are incredibly nutritious. They are packed with protein, fiber, and a variety of vitamins and minerals

Nuts may help you lose weight and reduce the risk of developing type 2 diabetes and heart disease.

Additionally, one large observational study noted that a low intake of nuts and seeds was potentially linked to an increased risk of death from heart disease, stroke, or type 2 diabetes.

3. Avoid ultra-processed foods

Ultra-processed foods are foods containing ingredients that are significantly modified from their original form. They often contain additives like added sugar, highly refined oil, salt, preservatives, artificial sweeteners, colors, and flavors as well (10Trusted Source).

Examples include:

Snack cakes

Fast food

Frozen meals

Canned foods

Chips

Ultra-processed foods are highly palatable, meaning they are easily overeaten, and activate reward-related regions in the brain, which can lead to excess calorie consumption and weight gain. Studies show that diets high in ultra-processed food can contribute to obesity, type 2 diabetes, heart disease, and other chronic conditions.

In addition to low quality ingredients like inflammatory fats, added sugar, and refined grains, they're usually low in fiber, protein, and micronutrients. Thus, they provide mostly empty calories.

4. Don't fear coffee

Despite some controversy over it, coffee is loaded with health benefits.

It's rich in antioxidants, and some studies have linked coffee intake to longevity and a reduced risk of type 2 diabetes, Parkinson's and Alzheimer's diseases, and numerous other illnesses

The most beneficial intake amount appears to be 3–4 cups per day, although pregnant people should limit or avoid it completely because it has been linked to low birth weight. However, it's best to consume coffee and any caffeine-based items in moderation. Excessive caffeine intake may lead to health issues like insomnia and heart palpitations. To enjoy coffee in a safe and healthy way, keep your intake to less than 4 cups per day and avoid high-calorie, high-sugar additives like sweetened creamer.

5. Eat fatty fish

Fish is a great source of high-quality protein and healthy fat. This is particularly true of fatty fish, such as salmon, which is loaded with anti-inflammatory omega-3 fatty acids and various other nutrients.

Studies show that people who eat fish regularly have a lower risk for several conditions, including heart disease, dementia, and inflammatory bowel disease.

6. Get enough sleep

The importance of getting enough quality sleep cannot be overstated.

Poor sleep can drive insulin resistance, can disrupt your appetite hormones, and reduce your physical and mental performance.

What's more, poor sleep is one of the strongest individual risk factors for weight gain and obesity. People who do not get enough sleep tend to make food choices that are higher in fat, sugar, and calories, potentially leading to unwanted weight gain.

7. Feed your gut bacteria

The bacteria in your gut, collectively called the gut microbiota, are incredibly important for overall health.

A disruption in gut bacteria is linked to some chronic diseases, including obesity and a myriad of digestive problems.

Good ways to improve gut health include eating probiotic foods like yogurt and sauerkraut, taking probiotic supplements — when indicated — and eating plenty of fiber. Notably, fiber serves as a prebiotic, or a food source for your gut bacteria.

8. Stay hydrated

Hydration is an important and often overlooked marker of health. Staying hydrated helps ensure that your body is functioning optimally and that your blood volume is sufficient.

Drinking water is the best way to stay hydrated, as it's free of calories, sugar, and additives.

Although there's no set amount that everyone needs per day, aim to drink enough so that your thirst is adequately quenched.

9. Don't eat heavily charred meats

Meat can be a nutritious and healthy part of your diet. It's very high in protein and a rich source of nutrients.

However, problems occur when meat is charred or burnt. This charring can lead to the formation of harmful compounds that may increase your risk for certain cancers.

When you cook meat, try not to char or burn it. Additionally limit your consumption of red and processed meats like lunch meats and bacon as these are linked to overall cancer risk and colon cancer risk.

10. Avoid bright lights before sleep

When you're exposed to bright lights — which contain blue light wavelengths — in the evening, it may disrupt your production of the sleep hormone melatonin.

Some ways to help reduce your blue light exposure is to wear blue light blocking glasses — especially if you use a computer or other digital screen for long periods of time — and to avoid digital screens for 30 minutes to an hour before going to bed.

This can help your body better produce melatonin naturally as evening progresses, helping you sleep better.

11. Take vitamin D if you're deficient

Most people do not get enough vitamin D. While these widespread vitamin D inadequacies are not imminently harmful, maintaining adequate vitamin D levels can help to optimize your health by improving bone strength, reducing symptoms of depression, strengthening your immune system, and lowering your risk for cance.

If you do not spend a lot of time in the sunlight, your vitamin D levels may be low.

If you have access, it's a great idea to have your levels tested, so that you can correct your levels through vitamin D supplementation if necessary.

12. Eat plenty of fruits and vegetables

Vegetables and fruits are loaded with prebiotic fiber, vitamins, minerals, and antioxidants, many of which have potent health effects.

Studies show that people who eat more vegetables and fruits tend to live longer and have a lower risk for heart disease, obesity, and other illnesses

13. Eat adequate protein

Eating enough protein is vital for optimal health, as it provides the raw materials your body needs to create new cells and tissues.

What's more, this nutrient is particularly important for maintenance of a

Moderate body weight.

High protein intake may boost your metabolic rate — or calorie burn — while making you feels full. It may also reduce cravings and your desire to snack late at night.

14. Get moving

Doing aerobic exercise, or cardio, is one of the best things you can do for your mental and physical health.

It's particularly effective at reducing belly fat, the harmful type of fat that builds up around your organs. Reduced belly fat may lead to major improvements in your metabolic health.

According to the Physical Activity Guidelines for Americans, we should strive for at least 150 minutes of moderate intensity activity each week.

15. Don't smoke or use drugs, and only drink in moderation

Smoking, harmful use of drugs and alcohol abuse can all seriously negatively affect your health.

If you do any of these actions, consider cutting back or quitting helping reduce your risk for chronic diseases.

There are resources available online — and likely in your local community, as well — to help with this. Talk with your doctor to learn more about accessing resources.

16. Use extra virgin olive oil

Extra virgin olive oil is one of the healthiest vegetable oils you can use. It's loaded with heart-healthy monounsaturated fats and powerful antioxidants that have anti-inflammatory properties.

Extra virgin olive oil may benefit heart health, as people who consume it have a lower risk for dying from heart attacks and strokes according to some evidence.

17. Minimize your sugar intake

Added sugar is extremely prevalent in modern food and drinks. A high intake is linked to obesity, type 2 diabetes, and heart disease.

The Dietary Guidelines for Americans recommend keeping added sugar intake below 10% of your daily calorie intake, while the World Health Organization recommends slashing added sugars to 5% or less of your daily calories for optimal health.

18. Limit refined carbs

Not all carbs are created equal.

Refined carbs have been highly processed to remove their fiber. They're relatively low in nutrients and may harm your health when eaten in excess. Most ultra-processed foods are made from refined carbs, like processed corn, white flour, and added sugars.

Studies show that a diet high in refined carbs may be linked to overeating, weight gain, and chronic diseases like type 2 diabetes and heart disease.

19. Lift heavy weights

Strength and resistance training are some of the best forms of exercises you can do to strengthen your muscles and improve your body composition.

It may also lead to important improvements in metabolic health, including improved insulin sensitivity — meaning your blood sugar levels are easier to manage — and increases in your metabolic rate, or how many calories you burn at rest.
If you do not have weights, you can use your own bodyweight or resistance bands to create resistance and get a comparable workout with many of the same benefits.
The Physical Activity Guidelines for Americans recommends resistance training twice per week.

20. Avoid artificial Tran's fats

Artificial Tran's fats are harmful, man-made fats that are strongly linked to inflammation and heart disease.
Avoiding them should be much easier now that they have been completely banned in the United States and many other countries. Note that you may still encounter some foods that contain small amounts of naturally occurring trans fats, but these are not associated with the same negative effects as artificial trans fats.

21. Use plenty of herbs and spices

There is a variety of herbs and spices at our disposal these days, more so than ever. They not only provide flavor but also may offer several health benefits as well.
For example, ginger and turmeric both have potent anti-inflammatory and antioxidant effects, which may help improve your overall health.
Due to their powerful potential health benefits, you should aim to include a wide variety of herbs and spices in your diet.

22. Nurture your social relationships

Social relationships — with friends, family, and loved ones you care about — are important not only for your mental well-being but also your physical health.
Studies show that people who have close friends and family are healthier and live much longer than those who do not.

23. Occasionally track your food intake

The only way to know exactly how many calories you eat is to weigh your food and use a nutrition tracker, as estimating your portion sizes and calorie intake is not unreliable.
Tracking can also provide insights into your protein, fiber, and micronutrient intake.

Though some studies have found a link between tracking calories and disordered eating tendencies, there is some evidence that suggests that people who track their food intake tend to be more successful at losing weight and maintaining their weight loss.

24. Get rid of excess belly fat

Excessive abdominal fat, or visceral fat, is a uniquely harmful type of fat distribution that is linked to an increased risk of cardiometabolic diseases like type 2 diabetes and heart disease.

For this reason, your waist size and waist-to-hip ratio may be much stronger markers of health than your weight.

Cutting refined carbs, eating more protein and fiber, and reducing stress (which can reduce cortisol, a stress hormone that triggers abdominal fat deposition) are all strategies that may help you get rid of belly fat.

25. Avoid restrictive diets

Diets are generally ineffective and rarely work well long term. In fact, past dieting is one of the strongest predictors for future weight gain.

This is because overly restrictive diets actually lower your metabolic rate, or the amount of calories you burn, making it more difficult to lose weight. At the same time, they also cause alterations to your hunger and satiety hormones, which make you hungrier and may cause strong food cravings for foods high in fat, calories, and sugar.

All of this is a recipe for rebound weight gain, or "yoyo" dieting.

Instead of dieting, try adopting a healthier lifestyle. Focus on nourishing your body instead of depriving it.

Weight loss should follow as you transition to whole, nutritious foods — which are naturally more filling while containing fewer calories than processed foods.

26. Eat whole eggs

Despite the constant back and forth about eggs and health, it's a myth that eggs are bad for you because of their cholesterol content. Studies show that they have minimal effect on blood cholesterol in the majority of people, and they're a great source of protein and nutrients.

Additionally, a review involving 263,938 people found that egg intake had no association with heart disease risk.

27. Meditate

Stress has a negative effect on your health. It can affect your blood sugar levels, food choices, susceptibility to sickness, weight, fat distribution, and more. For this reason, it's important to find healthy ways to manage your stress. Meditation is one such way, and it has some scientific evidence to support its use for stress management and improving health.

In one study involving 48 people with high blood pressure, type 2 diabetes, or both, researchers found that meditation helped lower LDL (bad) cholesterol and inflammation compared with the control group. Additionally, the participants in the meditation group reported improved mental and physical wellness.

The Role of Nutrition in Health

It is currently estimated that about half of all American adults have one or more preventable and diet-related chronic diseases, the most common of which include cardiovascular disease and type 2 diabetes. As the rate of these chronic diseases, which are often due to poor nutritional intake and physical inactivity, continues to climb, it is imperative that the role of nutrition in all aspects of health is fully understood.

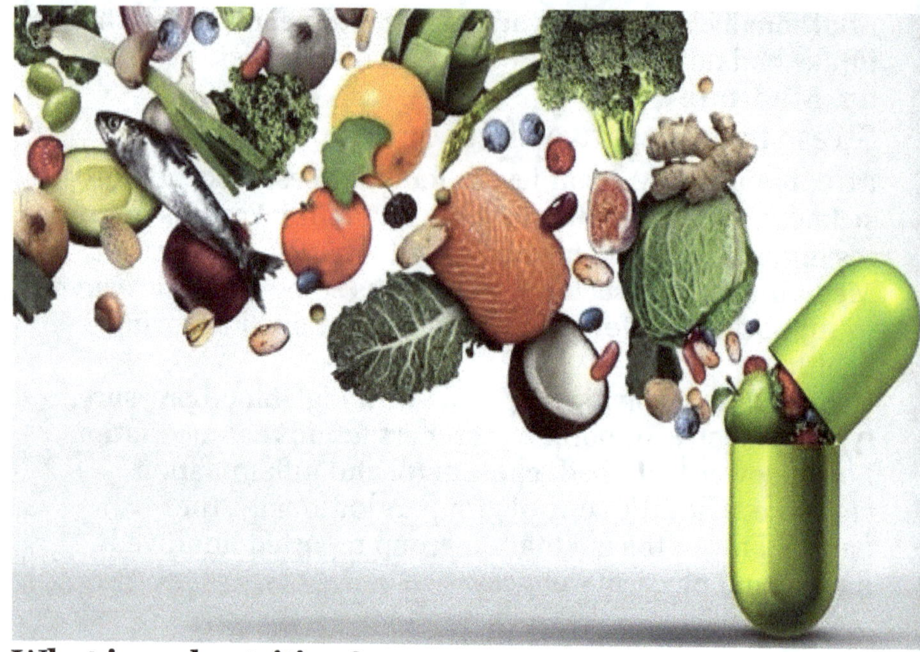

What is malnutrition?

According to the World Health Organization (WHO), malnutrition is a cellular imbalance that arises between the body's supply of nutrient and energy sources and the physical demand for these components. This imbalance can reduce the body's ability to grow and maintain adequate operation of various bodily functions. As a result, malnutrition can lead to a compromised health condition and increase an individual's risk of several different health conditions.

Malnutrition can be further classified into two broad forms, of which include undernutrition and micronutrient-related malnutrition. Under nutrition can be further divided into four forms that include wasting, stunting, underweight, and deficiencies in vitamins and minerals.

Comparatively, some of the different micronutrient-related malnutrition conditions include obesity and being overweight, diet-related non-communicable diseases, and an inadequate consumption of micronutrients.

Undernutrition

Wasting, which can also be defined as an individual with a low weight for their height, often occurs when said individual has recently lost a significant amount of waste. This severe weight loss can be due to a lack of food consumption, or as a result of an infectious disease, such as diarrhea.

Stunting, which is also known as low height-for-age, is a form of malnutrition that is due to chronic or recurrent undernutrition. Stunting is often associated with poor socioeconomic conditions, poor maternal health and nutrition, frequent illness and/or undernutrition in infants and young children.

Deficiencies in vitamin A, iron, iodine, and zinc are some of the most common outcomes of undernutrition. Vitamin A deficiency (VAD), for example, is the most common cause of preventable blindness and also increases an individual's risk of serious complications following an illness. In fact, it is currently estimated that VAD is responsible for 630,000 infectious deaths, particularly those due to measles, diarrhea, and malaria, each year.

A lack of both meat and plant consumption can lead to an iron deficiency, which can affect the body's ability to bind and transport oxygen, regulate cell growth and differentiation, and reduce immune function. Comparatively, an iodine deficiency can inhibit normal thyroid functions that are needed for the regulation of growth, development, and metabolic processes, as well as in the prevention of goiter and cretinism. Furthermore, iodine deficiency disorders (IDD) have also been associated with fetal loss, stillbirth, congenital anomalies, and impaired hearing capabilities.

Micronutrient-related nutrition

An individual who is obese or overweight is considered to be too heavy for his or her height. More specifically, a body mass index (BMI) for an individual who is overweight is typically over 25, whereas an obese individual will often have a BMI greater than 30. Since the early 2000s, abdominal obesity has affected about 50% of all American adults, with its prevalence increasing with age. It is currently estimated that 2.3 billion children and adults are overweight in the world.

The double burden of malnutrition is used to describe the paradox that exists between undernourishment and obesity. Although an obese individual may not appear to be malnourished, they often lack a diet that is rich in fruits, vegetables, whole grains and beans, all of which are necessary to maintain an adequate nutritional status.

In addition to increasing their risk of a number of health conditions such as cardiovascular diseases (CVD), diabetes and hypertension, obesity and malnutrition can also increase an individual's risk of experiencing various forms of cognitive impairment.

Tips for Improving Your Health

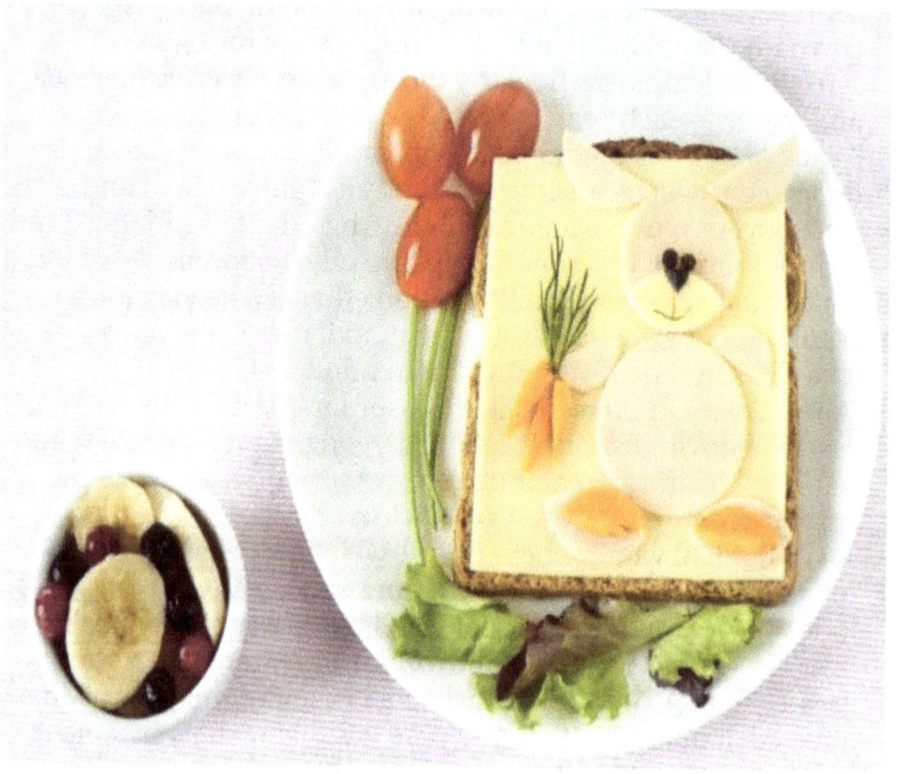

Good nutrition is one of the keys to a healthy life. You can improve your health by keeping a balanced diet. You should eat foods that contain vitamins and minerals. This includes fruits, vegetables, whole grains, dairy, and a source of protein. Ask yourself the following questions. If you answer yes to any of them, talk to your doctor about your health. You may need to improve your eating habits for better nutrition:

- Do you have a health problem or risk factor, such as high blood pressure, diabetes, or high cholesterol?

- Did your doctor tell you that you can improve your condition with better nutrition?

- Do diabetes, cancer, heart disease, or osteoporosis run in your family?

- Are you overweight?

- Do you have questions about what foods you should eat or whether you should take vitamins?

- Do you eat a lot of processed and fast foods?

- Do you think that you would benefit from seeing a registered dietitian or someone who specializes in nutrition counseling?

Path to improved health

It can be hard to change your eating habits. It helps to focus on small changes. Making changes to your diet may also be beneficial if you have diseases that can be worsened by the things you eat or drink. Symptoms from conditions such as kidney disease, lactose intolerance, and celiac disease can all benefit from changes in diet. Below are suggestions to improve your health. Be sure to stay in touch with your doctor so he or she knows how you are doing.

- Find the strengths and weaknesses in your current diet. Do you eat 4-5 cups of fruits and vegetables every day? Do you get enough calcium? Do you eat whole grain, high-fiber foods? If so, you're on the right track! Keep it up. If not, add more of these foods to your daily diet.

- Keep track of your food intake by writing down what you eat and drink every day. This record will help you assess your diet. You'll see if you need to eat more or less from certain food groups.

- Think about asking for help from a dietitian. He or she can help you follow a special diet, especially if you have a health issue.

Almost everyone can benefit from cutting back on unhealthy fat. If you currently eat a lot of fat, commit to cutting back and changing your habits. Unhealthy fats include things such as: dark chicken meat; poultry skin; fatty cuts of pork, beef, and lamb; and high-fat dairy foods (whole milk, butter, cheeses). Ways to cut back on unhealthy fats include:

- Bake, grill, or broil meat instead of frying it. Remove the skin before cooking chicken or turkey. Eat fish at least once a week.

- Reduce extra fat. This includes butter on bread, sour cream on baked potatoes, and salad dressings. Use low-fat or nonfat versions of these foods.

- Eat plenty of fruits and vegetables with your meals and as snacks.

- Read the nutrition labels on foods before you buy them. If you need help with the labels, ask your doctor or dietitian.

- When you eat out, be aware of hidden fats and larger portion sizes.

- Staying hydrated is important for good health. Drink zero- or low-calorie beverages, such as water or tea. Sweetened drinks add lots of sugar and calories to your diet. This includes fruit juice, soda, sports and energy drinks, sweetened or flavored milk, and sweetened iced tea.

Online Health and Nutrition Courses and Programs

Gain a better understanding of how food and nutrition impacts your health. Learn about how the three macronutrients, fat, carbohydrates and protein, are used to create energy for the body and how too much of these can lead to health problems. Wageningen University & Research in the Netherlands offers self-paced nutrition courses that go in-depth into the issues of obesity and malnutrition and the health problems associated with each. Understand the nutritional value and basic chemistry of vitamins and minerals and the role they play in the body. Learn about various food production strategies that can help combat malnutrition and reduce global hunger. Enroll in this 2-course program to understand nutrition facts and change the way you look at food.

Learn about the science behind fine dining with Science & Cooking: From Haute Cuisine to Soft Matter Science from Harvard University. In this free online course, students will learn about how molecules influence flavor, how heat impacts cooking and will engage in lab experiments in their own kitchens to learn first-hand the scientific principles behind cooking.

Have you ever been concerned about the risks of bacteria or pesticides in your food? Are you confused about how different meats need to be cooked to reduce the risk of illness? Learn how to separate fact from fiction in food safety with a free online course that gives an overview of food hazards along with ways to steer clear of them. Wageningen's free online course, Nutrition and Health: Food Risks, is a 10-week program that can help you stay healthy and safe in the kitchen or anywhere food is prepared or consumed.

Become a Nutritionist

Are you passionate about health and nutrition and would love to help educate others to develop healthy eating habits? A career as a nutritionist may be right for you. In addition to an undergraduate degree in food science, biology or similar field, nutritionists are often required to get a special nutrition certification in order to practice in the field. Enroll in online nutrition courses to learn more about this exciting career. Courses are free and self-paced so you can start learning today.

The Importance of Good Nutrition

Your daily food choices make a big difference in your health.

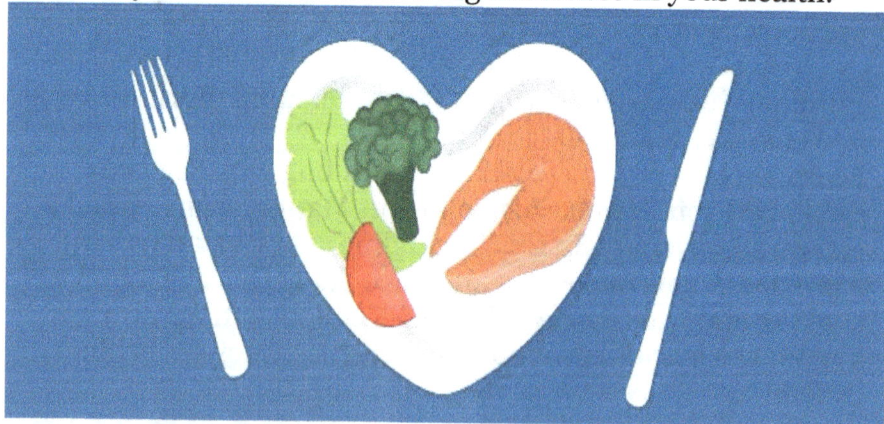

Why it's important

Most people know good nutrition and physical activity can help maintain a healthy weight. But the benefits of good nutrition go beyond weight. Good nutrition can help:

- Reduce the risk of some diseases, including heart disease, diabetes, stroke, some cancers, and osteoporosis

- Reduce high blood pressure

- Lower high cholesterol

- Improve your well-being

- Improve your ability to fight off illness

- Improve your ability to recover from illness or injury

- Increase your energy level

What is good nutrition?

Good nutrition means your body gets all the nutrients, vitamins, and minerals it needs to work its best. Plan your meals and snacks to include nutrient-dense foods that are also low in calories.

Tips for eating well

Eat plenty of fruit

To get the benefit of the natural fiber in fruits, you should eat fruit whole rather than as juices.

Eat plenty of vegetables

Eat a variety of colors and types of vegetables every day.

Eat plenty of whole grains

At least half of the cereals, breads, crackers, and pastas you eat should be made from whole grains.

Choose low fat or fat free milk

These provide calcium and vitamin D to help keep your bones strong.

Choose lean meats

Lean cuts of meat and poultry have less fat and fewer calories but are still good sources of protein.

Try other sources of protein
Try replacing meats and poultry with fish, beans, or tofu.
How to fix 5 common eating problems
As you age, you may lose interest in eating and cooking. Small changes can help you overcome some of the challenges to eating well.
1. Food no longer tastes good.
Try new recipes or adding different herbs and spices. Some medicines can affect your appetite or sense of taste - talk to your doctor.
2. Chewing difficulty.
Try softer foods like cooked vegetables, beans, eggs, applesauce, and canned fruit. Talk to your doctor or dentist if there is a problem with your teeth or gums.
3. Poor digestion.
Talk to your doctor or registered dietician to figure out which foods to avoid while still maintaining a balanced diet.
4. Eating alone.
Try dining out with family, friends, or neighbors. See if your local senior center hosts group meals.
5. Difficulty shopping or cooking.
Check with your local senior center for programs that can help you with shopping or preparing meals.

How good nutrition boosts your health

• Weight management
A lot of us mistakenly associate weight loss with fad diets, but eating a nutritious diet is really the best way to go about maintaining a healthy weight and at the same time attaining the necessary nutrients for healthy body function. Swapping unhealthy junk food and snacks out for nutritious food is the first step to keeping your weight within a healthy range relative to your body composition, without the need to jump on the fad-diet bandwagon.
• Protecting you from chronic diseases

Many chronic diseases such as type-2 diabetes and heart disease are caused by poor nutrition and obesity. With 1 in 9 Singaporeans suffering from diabetes, the emphasis on good nutrition is higher than ever. Taking a preventive approach with a whole food-based nutrition plan also reduces the risk of developing other related diseases such as kidney failure.

• **Strengthening your immune system**
Our immune system requires essential vitamins and minerals in order to function optimally. Eating a wholesome and varied diet ensures your immune system functions at peak performance and guards against illnesses and immunodeficiency problems.

• **Delaying the onset of ageing**
Certain types of food such as tomatoes and berries can increase vigour and improve cognitive performance, all the while protecting your body against the effects of ageing.

• **Supporting your mental well-being**
Eating the right foods can actually make you happier – nutrients such as iron and omega-3 fatty acids found in protein-rich food can boost your mood. This contributes to better overall mental well-being and protects you against mental health issues.

So, how does one build a sensible nutrition plan then? Healthy eating is all about eating balanced proportions of nutrient-rich foods from the various food groups, as well as adopting several healthy eating habits.

How to achieve good nutrition in your diet

Each food group provides different nutrients and benefits, so eating a balanced diet that includes foods from all five groups is essential. These are the different food groups that you should keep in mind.

1. Whole grains

Whole-grain foods such as brown rice and bread are forms of carbohydrates, specifically unrefined carbohydrates. They provide you with energy, healthy fiber, vitamins, minerals and antioxidants, and aid with digestion. For people who are diagnosed with coeliacs or those with non-coeliac gluten sensitivity, it's important that you include other carbohydrate alternatives to ensure that your abstinence from wheat doesn't cost you in terms of essential nutrients.

"Gluten-free carbohydrate alternatives include rice products, buckwheat (technically a pseudo cereal), quinoa and starchy vegetables (e.g., sweet potato, yam, pumpkin, corn)," says Ang Sin Hewed, Associate Sport Dietitian at Singapore Sport Institute. "As following a gluten-free diet may lead you to unknowingly cut out certain nutrients, it is recommended that you seek help from a registered dietitian."

2. Fruits and vegetables

Various forms of produce are rich sources of vitamins and minerals that help regulate body functions and protect it against chronic diseases. To get the most nutrients out of your fruits and vegetables, eat them whole – for example, eat whole fruits instead of having them juiced.

3. Protein

Protein is the primary nutrient responsible for building and repairing muscle tissue in the body. Animal meat is the most common source of protein, but there are also several plant-based options to choose from such as nuts and legumes. Individuals on plant-based diets should ensure that eat the right combination of plant protein to ensure that their dietary needs are adequately met.

4. Dairy

Dairy products are rich in important nutrients like calcium, potassium, phosphorus, vitamins A, D and B12. Foods like milk, yoghurt and cheese are great examples of dairy which can be found in practically every grocery store.

5. Fat and sugar

Dietary fat (such as the kind you get from fish and olive oil) is essential for good health as they regulate cholesterol levels in your body while promoting healthy cell function. Monounsaturated, polyunsaturated and saturated fat all play a role in this aspect of good health. On the other hand, the additional fat you often find in fried food should be minimized as they are largely polyunsaturated fat derived from processed vegetable oils such as soybean and rapeseed.

Due to their low threshold for oxidization, overconsumption of polyunsaturated fat can lead to inflammatory conditions and the formation of free radicals. Artificial trans-fat is also a strict "no-no". Sugar should also be limited – while the natural sugars present in fruits and whole grains are healthy, the refined sort you get with cakes and snacks can affect your weight and lead to metabolic diseases if consumed in excess. Apart from eating foods from the above-mentioned food groups, there are three other healthy eating habits to maintain in order to keep your nutrition plan on point.

• **Keep portion sizes regulated**

Managing portion sizes is all about ensuring that you are getting the right amounts of nutrients and calories from your food. Over-eating or under-eating deprives you of nutrients and can affect your weight, so always regulate your meal portions. When buying food, check out the serving sizes on the nutrition labels to see what amounts to a regular serving and how much it provides in terms of nutrients.

• **Priorities fresh food**

Fresh, whole foods are the ones you will derive maximum nutritional benefits from. Always go for foods in their purest, unprocessed form such as fresh fruits, vegetables and meat when possible. If you go with processed alternatives, pick those that have undergone simple changes such as dehydration and flash freezing to minimize nutrient loss. Also, keep an eye on the ingredients list to ensure that you're consuming as little additives with your food as possible.

• **Practice healthier seasoning habits**

Consider tempering your salt intake with other herbs and spices to add a new dimension of flavor to your food. For example, basil, garlic, paprika and cayenne can turn an ordinary chicken breast dish into a gastronomical delight! Salt is the most common food seasoning used in cooking, but too much sodium can lead to high blood pressure and hypertension, particularly with those who are already susceptible to said conditions.

Maintaining a nutritious eating plan is simple enough; evaluating whether it's nutritious enough can be straightforward as well. Just look out for five simple enough indicators of whether you are getting enough from your food.

Indicators of a nutritious diet

1. Body composition

A well-structured nutrition plan should allow an individual to maintain a healthy physique within acceptable body fat levels (18-24% for men and 25-31% for women). This also means that it should support metabolic health through a number of means, such as promoting healthy hormone function, insulin sensitivity and physical recovery.

2. Healthy cholesterol levels and blood pressure

Monitoring your cholesterol levels and blood pressure is crucial because having a healthy weight doesn't discount the possibility of issues in these areas. While dietary cholesterol doesn't have as much effect on blood cholesterol levels as we once thought, it can still be influenced by your overall dietary fat intake. On the other end, excessive sodium intake can lead to hyper-extension, of which one of the symptoms happens to be elevated blood pressure levels.

3. Healthy skin and hair

The condition of your skin and hair are good indicators of the quality of your nutrition. If you are getting enough nutrients, your skin should be firm, supple and of a rich hue rather than flaking and pale. Your hair should be smooth and strong rather than dry and brittle; unexplained hair loss is often a sign of malnutrition.

4. Sleep and energy levels
Getting the right amount of nutrients and calories will help
you stay energized due to its ability to promote restful sleep. If
you find yourself feeling sluggish, it could be a sign of either a
distinct lack of calories and/or nutrients, driving your body
into "starvation mode" which hampers its restorative
capabilities.

5. Regular bowel movements
Your bowel movements reflect whether you are getting
sufficient fiber from your diet, so if you find yourself being
constipated, load up on more fruits and vegetables to get your
digestive system going.

While these five indicators of a nutritious diet may give you're
a decent idea of how to go about achieving your nutrition
goals, getting the help of a certified nutritionist can help
improve your odds of success while avoiding the common
pitfalls.

Why you should consider seeing a nutritionist
• Advice and meal plans
When you're a busy working adult, planning your meals to
meet your nutritional requirements can be too much work. A
nutritionist can handle this easily and probably plan a more
nutritious meal than you can. You can also get advice on food
and nutrition, instead of searching through possibly unreliable
sources on the internet and endlessly questioning their
integrity.

• Adaptation
No battle plan survives the first contact, and the same goes for
nutrition plans. However, a well-trained nutritionist will know
exactly how and where to make adjustments to your eating
plan in order to get you back on track. From recently
discovered food allergies to accidental bingeing, it's all par for
the course to a nutritionist.

• Help you stick to your goal

It can be hard to work through diet-related problems alone. Having a nutritionist means you have someone to work through your problems and relapses with as well as someone to push you towards achieving your nutrition goals. Apart from diet-related advice, nutritionists can also offer emotional support when you are struggling to maintain the diet.

Picking the right nutritionist

If you've decided that seeing a nutritionist is a worthy investment, it's important to consider the different types of nutritionists. Not all nutritionists are equally qualified, so does a background check before you engage one. Some nutritionists are also registered dietitians who can help you create a tailor-made eating plan. Nutritionists who are not registered dietitians can usually only give advice in specific areas, such as sports nutrition.

There is yet another type of nutritionist called the holistic nutritionist. They focus on overall health and wellness, so if you have a specific health problem or goal to work towards to such as coping with a metabolic disorder, a holistic nutritionist may not be able to help as much. Furthermore, certifications for holistic nutritionists aren't as regulated so there's always the risk of being stuck with a lemon.

Whether or not it's to the advice of a professional or your inner voice, enjoying good nutrition is something that everyone should work towards. Good nutrition contributes heavily to your overall health and wellness and should never be skimped on. You can start your journey by joining our Active Health Coaches at Active Health Labs located island-wide for a fitness and health assessment to get the insights that will help you plan your nutrition plan better. From there on, it's upward and onward!

Benefits of healthy eating

A diversified, balanced and healthy diet will vary depending on:

- age

- gender

- lifestyle

- degree of physical activity

- cultural context

- locally available foods

- Dietary and food customs.

10 reasons why nutrition is important

Humans consume different types of foods each day. These foods comprise several nutritious values and most times, we do not even understand their benefits. A good nutrition plan is practiced by only a few people all around the world today. Many people are not informed of what benefits they tend to gain when they pay more attention to their nutrition plan. The food choices you make each day can affect your health, how you feel today, tomorrow, and also in the future.

It is necessary to note that good nutrition is an important aspect of living a healthy lifestyle. Usually, when good nutrition is combined with physical activity, it can help maintain a healthy weight, reduce your risk of chronic diseases (like cancer and heart diseases), and also promote your overall health.

Here are some of the reasons why nutrition is important today:

1. Good Nutrition Improves Well-Being

Eating a poor diet can reduce both mental and physical health. Eating healthy gives people the chance to be active in their daily lives. You need to ensure that your diet is full of complex carbohydrates, essential fats, vitamins and minerals. People who eat fresh fruits and vegetables report fewer cases of mental health issues. Once you can ensure that your diet comprises these nutrients, then you can be sure of enjoying the overall well-being of your body.

2. It is expensive to be unhealthy

Unhealthy foods can lead to conditions such as obesity or overweight. These conditions as well as others due to unhealthy diet plans can be quite expensive to control. According to research, billions of dollars can be saved yearly if people can maintain a healthy diet.

3. Helps You Manage a Healthy Weight

Once you start taking the necessary steps to eat healthily, you are definitely going to get the nutrients your body needs to stay, active, healthy, and strong. Your weight also will naturally be in check.

Janelle Hedonic, a Registered Dietician with Unity Point Clinic – Weight Loss, says this about nutrition: "There is no one diet, no diet pill and no surgery that lets people eat whatever they want and still expect weight loss and improved health. Maintaining a healthy diet and exercise program will be what is needed to achieve those goals. Use food for its purpose: Nourishment."

4. Maintains Your Immune System

The immune system is responsible for protecting the body against several diseases. Poor nutrition can make the immune system weak leaving the body prone to several attacks from bacteria, pathogens etc. By eating a well-balanced diet with fruits and vegetables, you can be sure that your immune system will be healthy.

5. Delays The Effect of Ageing

Although everyone is going to grow old at a certain point in life, the whole wrinkles, reduction in body side are some of the features of ageing. But this whole process can be delayed if we ensure a proper good diet plan and nutrition. Foods like tomatoes and berries improve the skin condition, making it firmer and also for cell regeneration of the skin.

6. Gives Your Body Energy

Carbohydrates, proteins and fats are found in most food we eat today and are responsible for giving the body energy. Carbohydrates are the vest category of food to eat for a prolonged supply of energy to the body. Eating good food means maintaining a proper consumption of a balanced diet which improves our nutrition plan.

7. Reduces the Risk of Chronic Diseases

Unhealthy eating can be the major cause of type 2 diabetes, especially in the younger generation according to the Centers for Disease Control and Prevention. It is important to teach our children and make it a culture for them on the importance of a good diet plan.

8. Healthy Eating Positively Affects Your Mood

Happier people tend to eat healthy while people that are sad tend to eat unhealthy foods. For instance, eating foods rich in protein, moderate in carbohydrates and low in fat will have a positive effect on mood. This is because it leaves an adequate supply of omega-3 fatty acids and iron.

9. Good Nutrition Increases Focus

Our daily lives are usually occupied by several activities that require our focus in order to get the best output. The kind of food we consume has an impact on the way we think generally. Eating fruits during the day keeps the mind healthy. It is advised that people avoid a high intake of fats as it can damage the brain.

10. Healthy Diets May Lengthen Your Life

The healthier you eat, the better you live. Just like we stated earlier, healthy foods can help delay ageing and as a result, might be able to increase your lifespan. Overeating should be avoided as it can cause more stress to the body during metabolism. Eating healthy food moderately is your best bet. Eating healthy might be quite expensive, but it is worth it when you have a good dietary plan not just for yourself but for your family.

Why is nutrition important to us?

Every food we consume contains important nutrition like proteins, carbohydrates, fats, vitamins, minerals, etc. Every nutrition plays a different role to keep our body healthy. Proteins:

Protein helps to build muscles and a strong immune system in our body. Proteins consist of amino acids. There are 22 varieties of amino acids. Our body fundamentally needs all these amino acids for better function. Protein is an abundant nutrient that builds new tissues and cures all damaged cells in our body. It helps in the formation of hormones and enzymes. Some protein sources are lentils, low-fat dairy products, tofu, nuts, seeds, peas, etc.

Carbohydrates:

Carbohydrates produce energy and help in the formation of cellular constituents. Carbohydrates are made of three compounds Carbon, Hydrogen, and Oxygen produced by plants. Carbohydrates don't cause any weight gain, unless like another food group. Simple carbohydrates and complex carbohydrates are the two different types of carbohydrates. Carbohydrates are the main reason for the production of ketones. Good examples of carbohydrates are bread, potatoes, pasta, soda, chips, cookies/biscuits, puddings, cakes, sugar, bananas, etc.

Fats:

Fat is extra energy and nutrient developed in the body. Fats are generally insoluble in water. Fat has 8 calories per gram. Fatty acids are naturally produced when dietary fats are digested. Fat is important for healthy skin and blood pressure regulation. Saturated fats and Unsaturated fats are the two different varieties of fats. Saturated fats are present in products like cream, butter, cheese, and some chocolates. Some of the unsaturated fats are sunflower, soybean, cardamom, and corn oils.

Vitamins:

A vitamin is an essential compound that plays an important role to make our body function properly. There are 12 vitamins necessary for our body. Some of them are vitamin A, vitamin B, vitamin C, vitamin D, vitamin E, vitamin K, vitamin B-6, and vitamin B-12. We receive most of these vitamins daily. Our body naturally has the tendency of producing vitamins like D and K.

Minerals:

Minerals help in the formation of body tissues. Minerals organize our immune system to work efficiently, but it doesn't prevent weight loss. Some important minerals are Calcium, Copper, Chloride, Chromium, Iron, Iron, Fluoride, and Iodine.

Eating the Right Foods for Exercise

Nutrition is important for fitness

Eating a well-balanced diet can help you get the calories and nutrients you need to fuel your daily activities, including regular exercise.

When it comes to eating foods to fuel your exercise performance, it's not as simple as choosing vegetables over doughnuts. You need to eat the right types of food at the right times of the day.

Get off to a good start

Your first meal of the day is an important one.

According to an article published in Harvard Health Letter, eating breakfast regularly has been linked to a lower risk of obesity, diabetes, and heart disease. Starting your day with a healthy meal can help replenish your blood sugar, which your body needs to power your muscles and brain.

Eating a healthy breakfast is especially important on days when exercise is on your agenda. Skipping breakfast can leave you feeling lightheaded or lethargic while you're working out.

Choosing the right kind of breakfast is crucial. Too many people rely on simple carbohydrates to start their day. A plain white bagel or doughnut won't keep you feeling full for long. In comparison, a fiber- and protein-rich breakfast may fend off hunger pangs for longer and provide the energy you need to keep your exercise going.

Follow these tips for eating a healthy breakfast:

- Instead of eating sugar-laden cereals made from refined grains, try oatmeal, oat bran, or other whole-grain cereals that are high in fiber. Then, throw in some protein, such as milk, yogurt, or chopped nuts.

- If you're making pancakes or waffles, replace some of the all-purpose flour with whole-grain options. Then, stir some cottage cheese into the batter.

- If you prefer toast, choose whole-grain bread. Then pair it with an egg, peanut butter, or another protein source.

Count on the right carbohydrates

Thanks to low-carb fad diets, carbohydrates have gotten a bad rap. But carbohydrates are your body's main source of energy. According to the Mayo Clinic, about 45 to 65 percent of your total daily calories should come from carbohydrates. This is especially true if you exercise.

Consuming the right kind of carbohydrates is important. Many people rely on the simple carbs found in sweets and processed foods. Instead, you should focus on eating the complex carbs found in whole grains, fruits, vegetables, and beans.

Whole grains have more staying power than refined grains because you digest them more slowly.

They can help you feel full for longer and fuel your body throughout the day. They can also help stabilize your blood sugar levels. Finally, these quality grains have the vitamins and minerals you need to keep your body running at its best.

Pack protein into your snacks and meals

Protein is needed to help keep your body growing, maintained, and repaired. For example, the University of Rochester Medical Center reports that red blood cells die after about 120 days.

Protein is also essential for building and repairing muscles, helping you enjoy the benefits of your workout. It can be a source of energy when carbohydrates are in short supply, but it's not a major source of fuel during exercise.

Adults need to eat about 0.8 grams of protein per day for every kilogram of their body weight, reports Harvard Health Blog. That's equal to about 0.36 grams of protein for every pound of body weight. Exercisers and older adults may need even more. Protein can come from:

- poultry, such as chicken and turkey

- red meat, such as beef and lamb

- fish, such as salmon and tuna

- dairy, such as milk and yogurt

- legumes, such as beans and lentils

- eggs

For the healthiest options, choose lean proteins that are low in saturated and trans fats. Limit the amount of red meat and processed meats that you eat.

Boost your fruit and vegetable intake

Fruits and vegetables are rich sources of natural fiber, vitamins, minerals, and other compounds that your body needs to function properly. They're also low in calories and fat. Aim to fill half your plate with fruits and veggies at every meal, recommends the United States Department of Agriculture.

Try to "eat the rainbow" by choosing fruits and veggies of different colors. This will help you enjoy the full range of vitamins, minerals, and antioxidants that the produce aisle has to offer.

Every time you go to the grocery store, consider choosing a new fruit or vegetable to try. For snacks, keep dried fruits in your workout bag and raw veggies in the fridge.

Choose healthy fats

Unsaturated fats may help reduce inflammation and provide calories.

While fat is a primary fuel for aerobic exercise, we have plenty stored in the body to fuel even the longest workouts. However, getting healthy unsaturated fats helps to provide essential fatty acids and calories to keep you moving.

Healthy options include:

- nuts

- seeds

- avocados

- olives

- oils, such as olive oil

Fuel up before exercise

When it comes to fueling up before or after a workout, it's important to achieve the right balance of carbs and protein. Pre-workout snacks that combine carbohydrates with protein can make you feel more energized than junk foods made from simple sugars and lots of fat.

Consider stocking your workout bag and refrigerator with some of these simple snacks:

Bananas

Bananas are full of potassium and magnesium, which are important nutrients to get on a daily basis. Eating a banana can help replenish these minerals while providing natural sugars to fuel your workout. For added protein, enjoy your banana with a serving of peanut butter.

Berries, grapes, and oranges

These fruits are all full of vitamins, minerals, and water. They're easy on your intestines, give you a quick boost of energy, and help you stay hydrated. Consider pairing them with a serving of yogurt for protein.

Nuts

Nuts are a great source of heart-healthy fats and also provide protein and essential nutrients. They can give you a source of sustained energy for your workout.

Pair them with fresh or dried fruit for a healthy dose of carbohydrates. However, test these options to see how they settle. High-fat foods can slow digestion, and they may make food sit in your stomach too long if your workout is coming up quickly.

Nut butter

Many grocery stores carry single-serving packets of peanut butter that don't require refrigeration and can be easily stored in a gym bag. For a tasty protein-carbohydrate combo, you can spread peanut butter on:

- an apple

- a banana

- whole-grain crackers

- a slice of whole-grain bread

If you don't like peanut butter, try almond butter, soy butter, or other protein-rich alternatives.

Don't cut too many calories

If you're trying to lose weight or tone your body, you may be tempted to cut a ton of calories from your meals. Cutting calories is a key part of weight loss, but it's possible to go too far.

Weight loss diets should never leave you feeling exhausted or ill. Those are signs that you're not getting the calories you need for good health and fitness.

According to the National Heart, Lung, and Blood Institute Trusted Source, a diet containing 1,200 to 1,500 daily calories is suitable for most women who are trying to lose weight safely. A diet with 1,500 to 1,800 daily calories is appropriate for most men who are trying to shed excess pounds.

If you're very active or you don't want to lose weight while getting fit, you may need to eat more calories. Talk to your doctor or a dietitian to learn how many calories you need to support your lifestyle and fitness goals.

Balance is key

As you settle into an active lifestyle, you'll probably discover which foods give you the most energy and which have negative effects. The key is learning to listen to your body and balancing what feels right with what's good for you.

Follow these tips:

- Aim to make breakfast a part of your routine.

- Choose complex carbohydrates, lean protein sources, healthy fats, and a wide variety of fruits and veggies.

- Stock your fridge and gym bag with healthy workout snacks.

The right balance of carbohydrates, protein, and other nutrients can help fuel your exercise routine.

Nutrition tips for better health and longevity

Good nutrition is a critical part of health and development. According to the World Health Organization (WHO), better nutrition is related to improved health at all ages, a lower risk of diseases, and longevity.

Nutrition tips for diet

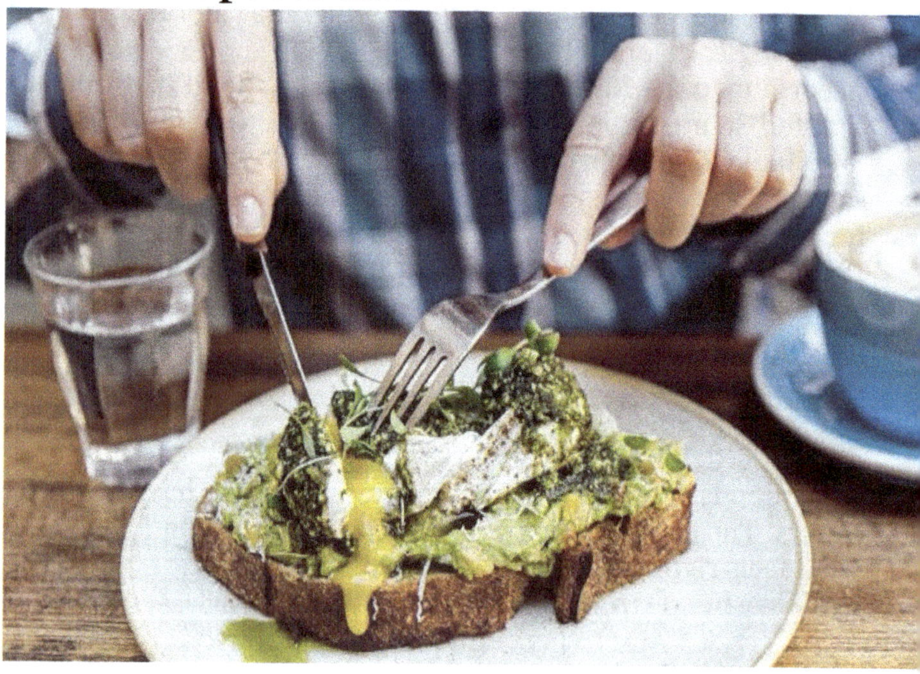

Following these nutrition tips will help a person make healthy food choices.

1. Include protein with every meal

Including some protein with every meal can help balance blood sugar.

Some studies suggest higher protein diets can be beneficial for type 2 diabetes.

Other research indicates balancing blood sugar can support weight management and cardiovascular health.

2. Eat oily fish

According to omega-3 fatty acids in oily fish are essential for cell signaling, gene expression, and brain and eye development.

Some studies indicate that omega-3 fatty acids can reduce the risk of cardiovascular disease.

Other research suggests the anti-inflammatory properties of omega-3 may effectively manage the early stages of degenerative diseases such as Alzheimer's disease and Parkinson's disease.

3. Eat whole grains

The American Heart Association (AHA) recommend people eat whole grains rather than refined grains.

Whole grains contain nutrients such as B vitamins, iron, and fiber. These nutrients are essential for body functions that include carrying oxygen in the blood, regulating the immune system, and balancing blood sugar.

4. Eat a rainbow

The saying 'eat a rainbow' helps remind people to eat different colored fruits and vegetables.

Varying the color of plant foods means that someone gets a wide variety of antioxidants beneficial o health, for example, carotenoids and anthocyanins.

5. Eat your greens

Dark green leafy vegetables are a great source of nutrition, according to the Department of Agriculture (USDA).

Leafy greens are rich in vitamins, minerals, and antioxidants. The USDA suggest that folate in leafy greens may help protect against cancer, while vitamin K helps prevent osteoporosis.

6. Include healthful fats

People should limit their intake of saturated fats while avoiding trans fats, according to the USDA.

A person can replace these fats with unsaturated fats, which they can find in foods such as avocado, oily fish, and vegetable oils.

7. Use extra virgin olive oil

As part of the Mediterranean diet, extra virgin olive oil has benefits to the heart, blood pressure, and weight, according to a 2018 health report.

A person can include extra virgin olive oil in their diet by adding it to salads or vegetables or cooking food at low temperatures.

8. Eat nuts

According to the AHA eating one serving of nuts daily in place of red or processed meat, French fries, or dessert may benefit health and prevent long-term weight gain.

The AHA suggests that Brazil nuts, in particular, may help someone feel fuller and stabilize their blood sugar.

9. Get enough fiber

According to the AHA fiber can help improve blood cholesterol levels and lower the risk of heart disease, obesity, and type 2 diabetes.

People can get enough fiber in their diet by eating whole grains, vegetables, beans, and pulses.

10. Increase plant foods

Research suggests that plant-based diets may help prevent overweight and obesity. Doctors associate obesity with many diseases.

According to some studies, including more plant foods in the diet could reduce the risk of developing diseases such as diabetes and cardiovascular disease.

11. Try beans and pulses

Beans and pulses are a good source of protein for people on a plant-based diet. However, those who eat meat can eat them on a few meat-free days a week.

Beans and pulses also contain beneficial fiber, vitamins, and minerals.

Some research even says pulses may help people feel fuller and lose weight.

Nutrition tips for what to drink

Drinking plenty of healthy fluids has numerous health benefits. Health experts recommend these tips:

12. Drink water

Drinking enough water every day is good for overall health and can help manage body weight, according to the Centers for Disease Control and Prevention (CDC).

Drinking water can prevent dehydration, which can be a particular risk for older adults.

If someone does not like plain water, they can add some citrus slices and mint leaves to increase the appeal or drink herbal teas.

13. Enjoy coffee

A 2017 study suggests that moderate coffee consumption of 3–5 cups a day can reduce the risk of:

- type 2 diabetes

- Alzheimer's disease

- Parkinson's disease

- cardiovascular diseases

According to the same review, the recommended amount reduces to 2 cups per day for pregnant and lactating people.

14. Drink herbal teas

According to research catechism in green, black, and other herbal teas may have antimicrobial properties.

Herbal teas, such as mint, chamomile, and rooibos, are caffeine-free and help keep someone hydrated throughout the day.

Nutrition tips for foods and drinks to avoid

It is important to cut back on food and drink that may have harmful health consequences. For example, a person may want to:

15. Reduce sugar

According to research dietary sugar, dextrose, and high fructose corn syrup may increase the risk of cardiovascular disease and metabolic syndrome.

People should look out for hidden sugars in foods that manufacturers label as names ending in "-use," for example, fructose, sucrose, and glucose.

Natural sugars, such as honey and maple syrup, could also contribute to weight gain if someone eats them too often.

16. Drink alcohol in moderation

Dietary Guidelines for Americans recommend that if someone consumes alcohol, it should be in moderation.

They advise up to one drink per day for females and up to two drinks per day for males.

Excessive drinking increases the risk of chronic diseases and violence, and over time, can impair short and long-term cognitive function.

17. Avoid sugary drinks

The CDC associate frequently drinking sugary drinks with:

- weight gain and obesity

- type 2 diabetes

- heart disease

- kidney disease

- non-alcoholic liver disease

- tooth decay and cavities

- gout, a type of arthritis

People should limit their consumption of sugary drinks and preferably drink water instead.

18. Eat less red and processed meat

A large prospective study in the British Medical Journal indicates that U.S. adults eating more red and processed meat had higher mortality rates.

Participants who swapped meat for other protein sources, such as fish, nuts, and eggs, had a lower risk of death in the eight-year study period.

19. Avoid processed foods

According to a review in Nutrients, eating ultra-processed foods can increase the risk of many diseases, including cancer, irritable bowel syndrome, and depression.

People should instead consume whole foods and avoid foods with long lists of processed ingredients.

Other good health habits

There are several steps a person can take to improve their health in addition to consuming healthful foods and drinks.

20. Support your micro biome

A 2019 review in Nutrients suggests that a high quality, balanced diet supports microbial diversity and can influence the risk of chronic diseases.

The authors indicate that including vegetables and fiber are beneficial to the microbiome. Conversely, eating too many refined carbohydrates and sugars is detrimental.

21. Consider a vitamin D supplement

The recommended dietary allowance for vitamin D is 15 micrograms or 600 international units per day for adults. Many people get some of their vitamin D from sunlight, while it is also in some foods.

People with darker skin, older adults, and those who get less exposure to sunlight — such as during winter or in less sunny climates — may need to take a vitamin D supplement.

22. be aware of portion size

Being aware of portion sizes can help people manage their weight and diet.

The USDA has helpful information about portion sizes for different food patterns.

People can adapt the guidelines to suit their cultural or personal preferences.

23. Use herbs and spices

Using herbs and spices in cooking can liven up a meal and have additional health benefits.

A 2019 review suggests that the active compounds in ginger may help prevent oxidative stress and inflammation that occurs as part of aging.

Curcumin in turmeric is anti-inflammatory and may have protective effects on health, according to research.

Garlic has many benefits including anti-inflammatory, antimicrobial, and antioxidant properties.

24. Give your body a rest by fasting

Intermittent fasting involves not eating either overnight or some days of the week. This may reduce energy intake and can have health benefits.

According to a 2020 review intermittent fasting may improve blood pressure, cholesterol levels, and heart health.

25. Keep a food journal

The American Society for Nutrition say that keeping a food journal can help people track calories, see how much they are eating, and recognize food habits.

Keeping a food journal could help someone who wants to maintain a moderate weight or eat a more healthful diet.

Apps, such as MyFitnessPal, can also help someone achieve their goals.

26. Wash fruits and vegetables

Raw fruits and vegetables can contain harmful germs that could make someone sick, according to the CDC. They advise that Salmonella, E.coli, and listeria cause a large percentage of U.S. foodborne illness.

Always wash fresh produce when eating them raw.

27. Do not microwave in plastic containers

Research suggests that microwaving food in plastic containers can release phthalates, which can disrupt hormones.

Experts recommend heating food in glass or ceramic containers that are microwave safe.

28. Eat varied meals

Many people eat the same meals regularly. Varying foods and trying different cuisines can help someone achieve their required nutrient intake.

This can be particularly helpful when trying to eat a broader range of vegetables or protein.

29. Eat mindfully

In a 2017 study mindful eating helped adults with obesity eat fewer sweets and manage their blood glucose.

Another study suggests mindfulness can bring greater awareness to food triggers and habits in people with diabetes.

Here are a few effective and tested ways that can help you improve your wellbeing:

1. Take Proper Sleep:

It may seem to be the most common advice but trust me most of the people don't follow the basic strep towards their overall wellbeing. Our body needs proper sleep and rest to heal and renew the energy to function properly. This healing is essential for physical and mental activity throughout the day. Sufficient sleep regulates the hormones that are directly related to our mood and emotions. Most often when you feel an irritated or emotional imbalance, chances are high that your body lacks in taking enough sleep. An adult body needs nearly 6 to 7 hours of sleep per day. So, make sure you take enough sleep.

2. Eat a Balanced Diet:

Sleep alone is not going to give you the required benefits. You need to eat a healthy and balanced diet and ensure your body receives enough amount of nutrition. The food you consume determines how healthy your inner system is. Moreover, it also helps in determining your emotional health and mental illnesses such as depression.

When your body lacks essential nutrients, it leads to serious health problems. Moreover, you end up facing emotional distress and anxiety. Health and wellness experts suggest that you should eat fruits and vegetables in sufficient amount. Moreover, eating nuts and lentil also strengthens your heart. Try to avoid caffeine, sugar and processed food as much as possible.

3. Expose Your Body to Sunlight:

Vitamin D deficiency leads to several problems such and Seasonal Affective Disorder or SAD. When you are exposed to sunlight, it causes the release of endorphins also called 'happiness hormones' that is responsible for the productivity of the brain.

So, take some time out of your routine and spend some time in sunlight. But makes sure you wear sunblock to prevent sunburn.

4. Deal with Stress:

Although it is difficult to avoid stress nowadays, however, it is definitely possible to deal with it. It is very important to learn to deal with stress in a smart and effective way. For that, try to avoid the situations that cause stress. If your stress is unmanageable, note down the causes of stress as well as what actions can you take to improve your reaction, mood, and even situation?

5. Exercise Daily:

When you remain physically active and exercise daily, your blood flow improves in your entire body. With the increased blood flow, the number of oxygen increases and you feel more energetic, fresh and mentally active.

Exercises and physical activities are more important if you are an office worker. Exercise not only ensures our body remains fit but also keeps your mind healthy as well. You don't have to join expensive gyms for that. A simple walk with your pet or daily morning walk is more than sufficient. The important thing is to make it a daily habit.

In addition to your mental health, exercise strengthens your bones and muscles that prevent you from a different type of personal injuries during a workout or running your daily errands.

6. Stay Away from Smoking and Alcohol:

If you keep drinking and smoking, no matter how much you spend on your health and how hard you try, your efforts are going to be wasted.

Quit smoking and drinking to ensure you lead a healthy life.

7. Be Social, as Much as You Can:

Isolation and lack of communication are the two biggest reasons for depression, mental and physical illnesses. No matter how busy your family and work life are, try to dedicate some time to friends and socialize with them.

A man cannot stay healthy without interacting with other people. Communicating with others lowers the stress level. If you have heard of laughter therapy, it also has the same purpose to reduce the stress in which you laugh with other people. Everyone needs acceptance and friendship that is fulfilled only when you socialize with others.

8. Find and Practice New Hobbies:

Hobby helps us keep busy and engaged. When you have an interest in some activities and enjoy doing them, you take healthy steps to improve your emotional wellbeing. It also keeps the work and daily life's pressure off your brain. Finding new hobbies is great for strengthening your brain and boosts your mood.

9. Learn to Live in the Present:

The biggest reason for experiencing mood swings, depression and anxiety is when a person remains stuck in past events. Negative self-talking such as 'why people did this to me' steal not only the happiness but make the person miss opportunities that the present moment tires to offer.

7 Tips to Improve Health and Wellness

Sustainability relies on actively improving within the different components of wellness. These tips can help nurture an ongoing basis.

1. Eat Whole Foods

Diet tends to be primarily viewed to impact physical health. However, food has a well-understood link between food and mental health, including boosting memory and improving mood.

A natural way to ensure adequate nutrients is by consuming whole foods rather than boxed and processed products. Balancing the diet with whole grains, fruits and veggies, lean and plant-based proteins, and healthy fats.

Utilizing bistro is also a sure way to include whole foods in the diet. Each meal is balanced with adequate protein, complex carbohydrates and fiber, and healthy fat to support a healthy weight and weight loss. All meals also nourish the body for optimal health while alleviating the stress of meal prep.

2. Exercise Regularly

Exercise stimulates a healthy mind and body, and the American Heart Association recommends at least 150 minutes of physical activity weekly. Regular exercise helps lower blood pressure, manage weight, boost mental health, amongst other benefits.

Also break away from the monotony of a structured workout regimen, as the highest importance is dismissing a sedentary lifestyle. Increase activity in your day by walking the dog, hiking with friends, and taking the steps over an elevator. Walking and biking whenever possible also not only emboldens both physical and mental health but supports environmental wellness by reducing fuel emission.

(And not to mention, saving on gas money!

3. Embrace Mental Exercises, Too

Most people do not consider mental exercises when they are trying to get fit physically. However, these types of activities can actually help you achieve your goals more sufficiently and boost brainpower!

Tackling daily brain exercises - think puzzles, learning new skills, etc. - helps support intellectual wellness. Practicing yoga or other combinations of mental and physical activities can help promote a better attitude towards weight loss.

4. Achieve Quality Sleep

Sleep is important for your mind and body, as adequate and sufficient sleep:

• Strengthens memory and concentration
• Lowers stress intensities
• Increases daily energy
• Diminishes cravings
• Regulates hunger levels

Sleep to such benefits by taking power naps as needed and getting a full night's rest on a regular basis. The National Sleep Foundation encourages healthy adults to sleep seven to nine hours of quality on a nightly basis.

If struggling to achieve the recommended hours of sleep each night, create a bedtime routine by:

• Staying consistent with bedtimes
• Powering down from electronics
• Evaluating and optimizing your room environment
• Practicing relaxation techniques

If still struggling with getting quality shuteye, consider consulting with a sleep specialist or another care provider. They can not only offer additional advice but ensure a sleep disorder is not impeding on getting adequate sleep.

5. Take a Day of Rest

In addition to achieving adequate sleep on a nightly basis, allow yourself days of rest and recovery.

Make sure to take one day out of the week to do something spontaneous or plan out a weekend trip you can look forward to. Doing so makes the whole "dieting" process more enjoyable - and life should be enjoyed!

Even if you cannot get away every weekend, make sure you do small things that you love on your day off. This could be as simple as going for a leisurely stroll, taking a walk in the park, or spending an evening relaxing to a movie.

6. Bask in Social Support

Social circles and support networks are invaluable for overall well-being and a sense of purpose.

A 75-year-old study discovered good relationships keep us happier and healthier, though the data truly is not so surprising. We as humans need to feel connected to others is one of our basic needs that need to be met.

Form and turn to your strongest supporters, including family members, friends, neighbors, and coworkers. Likewise, get them involved in your wellness journey by inviting them over for a home-cooked meal or exercise class.

7. Enjoy the Journey

One can make a target weight loss and health goal. However, sustainability relies on actively going through the different components of wellness.

Do not feel overwhelmed with large feats alone. Instead, take on small tasks, re-strategize as needed, and surround yourself with positive people. Also, embrace the journey and enjoy the process of achieving personal fulfillment and wellness!

Simple Ways to Improve Your Health and Wellness

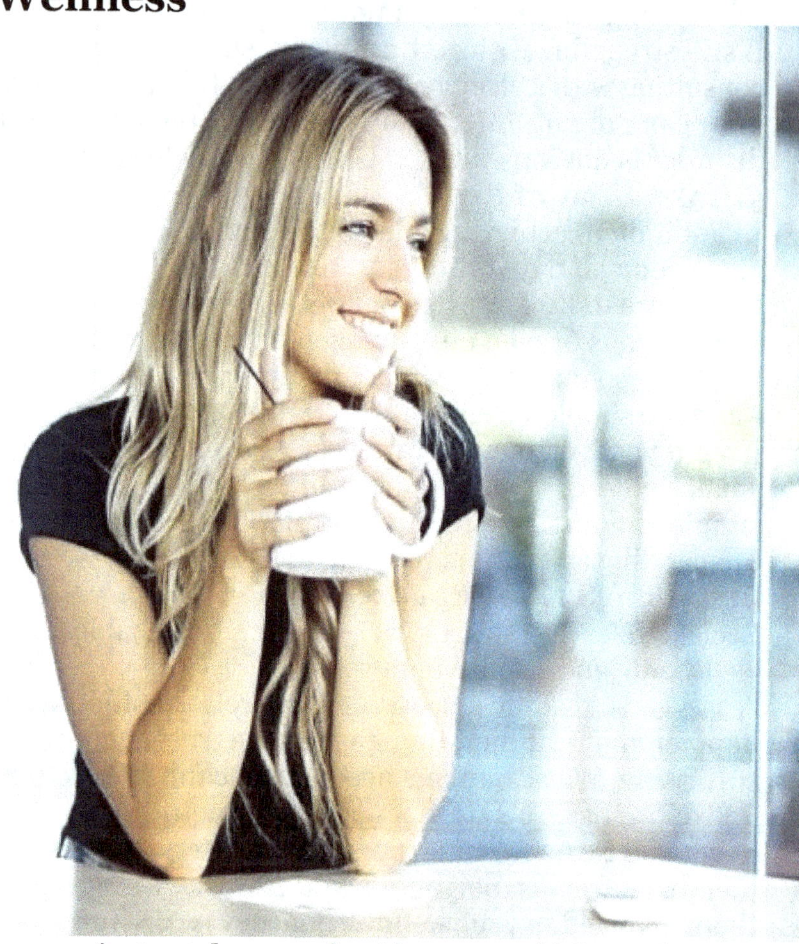

Have you ever just sat down and said to yourself, "I need to become happier and healthier." Seems like a pretty vague statement, doesn't it?

When you take on such a huge, and extremely vague, goal –
you will most likely fail. This is not because you don't have
what it takes to achieve this lifestyle; but having such big and
broad goals can be very intimidating.

The journey to becoming a healthier and happier individual is
just that, a journey. No single task will be able to accomplish
this goal. You need to accomplish small, achievable milestones
every day.

Here are 20 samples, and realistic, things you can do to
improve your health and wellness.

1. Drink More Water

Aim to drink 60oz of water every day. Try infusing your water
with fruits and veggies to make it less bland.

2. Get More Sleep

You should be getting 7-9 hours of GOOD sleep every night.
Having trouble sleeping? Before bedtime try drinking
chamomile tea, turning off all electronic devices, doing light
stretching or yoga, or taking a relaxing bubble bath.

3. Walk It Out

The average person should aim for 10,000 steps throughout
the entire day. If you have a desk job, get up every 30 minutes
to walk around the office or use your lunch hour for exercise.
Also try these awesome office workouts!

4. Stretch

Studies are finding that stretching can improve your health,
wellbeing, and quality of life. A lack of flexibility can lead to
high blood sugar, sore muscles, and stiff arteries.

5. Eat Breakfast

A lot of people make dinner their biggest meal of the day,
when it should be breakfast! Eating a healthy breakfast filled
with fiber and protein will boost metabolism, provide energy
throughout the day, and can improve focus. (Watch out for
those sugary cereals though!)

6. Meditate

You don't need to sit in a room for an hour to reap the benefits
of meditation. Simply take 5-10 minutes every day to clear
your mind and be one with yourself.

Meditation can decrease anxiety, increase creativity, improve immune system, lower blood pressure, decrease muscle tension, improve headaches, aid in problem solving, provide self-discovery, and increase serotonin which improves overall mood and behavior.

7. Cook Meals

A simple way to become healthier is making your own meals and eating at home. Restaurant food might be yummy, but it is filled with unwanted sodium, sugar, and bad fats.

8. Friends and Family Time

Spend more time with friends and family and your health and happiness will start to improve. Studies have shown that human interaction, especially with good friends and loved ones, will increase mood and decrease anxiety and depression.

9. Wash Your Sheets

The unappealing truth is that dust mites, dead skin cells, and other grimes love to sleep with you at night. So make sure you are cleaning your sheets and pillowcases every 1-2 weeks to avoid sickness and other health issues.

10. Clean your Dish Sponge

According to Charles Gerber, PhD, a microbiologist at the University of Arizona, "About 15 percent of sponges contain bacteria that can make you ill." Make sure you are cleaning your sponge at least once a week. Simply throw it in the dishwasher!

11. Use Technology

Use fitness trackers or health apps to monitor your activity level and overall health. These apps can track physical activity (like your amount of steps), sleep patterns, water intake, heart-rate, and much more!

12. Smile More

As they say, it takes more muscles to frown than to smile. Studies have shown that the act of simply smiling can instantly increase mood. Want a super boost? Laugh more too!

13. Go Outdoors

Being outdoors can increase mood, lower stress levels, boost creativity, and improve immune system.

Fresh air is full of satisfying negative ions, which can boost oxygen flow to the brain. Sunlight causes the body to make vitamin D, which is essential for bone health. About 20-25 minutes in sunlight should do the trick! Make sure you are wearing SPF to shield yourself from harmful UV rays.

14. Omega-3s

Consuming more omega-3s can reduce inflammation, combat depression and anxiety, improve memory, and increase mood. Some great sources of omega-3s are salmon, tuna, nuts, flax seeds, hemp seeds, and leafy greens.

15. Get Organized

Stress is one of the biggest obstacles to living a happy and healthy lifestyle. Having a disorganized desk, messy bedroom, and constantly missing important dates and appointments can cause a tremendous increase in stress levels.

Take 10-15 minutes every day to organize things at work, at home, and go over to-do lists. You will be shocked by how much your stress level decreases when you can actually find things, remember things, and not have clutter taking over your life.

16. Pay it Forward

Volunteering or performing simple selfless gestures is amazing for your health and wellness. Helping others is much more rewarding than any other material good – it's truly priceless! Want to start feeling healthier and happier? Give back!

17. Drink Tea

We recommend drinking green tea because there are so many health benefits!

Green tea can fight cancer, lower cholesterol, increase metabolism, detoxify your body, improve dental health, strengthen nervous system, and reduce depression, control blood glucose levels, and so much more!

Aim for at least one cup of green tea a day.

18. Set Goals

Setting goals (and writing them down) is great way to stay on task and keep moving forward and give you a sense of purpose. Set realistic goals that will help enhance all aspects of your life.

19. Wake Up Earlier

There are many benefits to waking up earlier!

Your day starts on a positive note, you won't feel rushed, you'll have time to eat a hearty breakfast, you can work out before work, and you can even watch the sunrise (bonus!).

20. Practice Yoga

Yoga is one of our favorite ways to improve health and wellness!

Participating in yoga can improve stiff muscles, improve breathing, mend posture, decrease blood pressure, improve sleep, help body aches, lower stress levels, and increase flexibility.

Path to improved health

Eat healthy.

What you eat is closely linked to your health. Balanced nutrition has many benefits. By making healthier food choices, you can prevent or treat some conditions. These include heart disease, stroke, and diabetes. A healthy diet can help you lose weight and lower your cholesterol, as well.

Get regular exercise.

Exercise can help prevent heart disease, stroke, diabetes, and colon cancer. It can help treat depression, osteoporosis, and high blood pressure. People who exercise also get injured less often. Routine exercise can make you feel better and keep your weight under control. Try to be active for 30 to 60 minutes about 5 times a week. Remember, any amount of exercise is better than none.

Lose weight if you're overweight.

Many Americans are overweight. Carrying too much weight increases your risk for several health conditions. These include:

- high blood pressure

- high cholesterol

- type 2 diabetes

- heart disease

- stroke

- some cancers

- gallbladder disease

Being overweight also can lead to weight-related injuries. A common problem is arthritis in the weight-bearing joints, such as your spine, hips, or knees. There are several things you can try to help you lose weight and keep it off.

Protect your skin.

Sun exposure is linked to skin cancer. This is the most common type of cancer in the United States. It's best to limit your time spent in the sun. Be sure to wear protective clothing and hats when you are outside. Use sunscreen year-round on exposed skin, like your face and hands. It protects your skin and helps prevent skin cancer. Choose a broad-spectrum sunscreen that blocks both UVA and UVB rays. It should be at least an SPF 15. Do not sunbathe or use tanning booths.

Practice safe sex.

Safe sex is good for your emotional and physical health. The safest form of sex is between 2 people who only have sex with each other. Use protection to prevent sexually transmitted diseases (STDs). Condoms are the most effective form of prevention. Talk to your doctor if you need to be tested for STDs.

Don't smoke or use tobacco.

Smoking and tobacco use are harmful habits. They can cause heart disease and mouth, throat, or lung cancer. They also are leading factors of emphysema and chronic obstructive pulmonary disease (COPD). The sooner you quit, the better.

Limit how much alcohol you drink.

Men should have no more than 2 drinks a day. Women should have no more than 1 drunk a day. One drink is equal to 12 ounces of beer, 5 ounces of wine, or 1.5 ounces of liquor. Too much alcohol can damage your liver. It can cause some cancers, such as throat, liver, or pancreas cancer. Alcohol abuse also contributes to deaths from car wrecks, murders, and suicides.

5 Simple Rules for Amazing Health

Following a healthy lifestyle often seems incredibly complicated.
Advertisements and experts all around you seem to give conflicting advice.
However, leading a healthy life doesn't need to be complicated. To gain optimal health, lose weight and feel better every day, all you need to do is follow these 5 simple rules.

1. Do Not Put Toxic Things into Your Body
Many things' people put in their bodies are downright toxic. Some, such as cigarettes, alcohol and abusive drugs, are also highly addictive, making it hard for people to give them up or avoid them.
If you have a problem with one of these substances, then diet and exercise are the least of your worries.
While alcohol is fine in moderation for those who can tolerate it, tobacco and abusive drugs are bad for everyone.
But an even more common problem today is eating unhealthy, disease-promoting junk foods.
If you want to gain optimal health, you need to minimize your consumption of these foods.
Probably the single most effective change you can make to improve your diet is to cut back on processed, packaged foods. This can be tough because many of these foods are designed to be extremely tasty and very hard to resist.
When it comes to specific ingredients, added sugars are among the worst. These include sucrose and high-fructose corn syrup. Both can wreak havoc on your metabolism when consumed in excess, though some people can tolerate moderate amounts.

In addition, it's a good idea to avoid all trans fats, which are found in some types of margarine and packaged baked foods.

2. Lift Things and Move Around

Using your muscles is extremely important for optimal health. While lifting weights and exercising can certainly help you look better, improving your appearance is really just the tip of the iceberg.

You also need to exercise to ensure your body, brain and hormones function optimally.

Lifting weights lowers your blood sugar and insulin levels, improves cholesterol and lowers triglycerides.

It also raises your levels of testosterone and growth hormones, both associated with improved well-being.

What's more, exercise can help reduce depression and your risk of various chronic diseases, such as obesity, type 2 diabetes, heart disease, Alzheimer's and many more.

Additionally, exercise may help you lose fat, especially in combination with a healthy diet. It doesn't just burn calories, but also improves your hormone levels and overall body function.

Fortunately, there are many ways to exercise. You don't need to go to a gym or own expensive workout equipment.

It's possible to exercise for free and in the comfort of your own home. Just do a search on Google or YouTube for "bodyweight workouts" or "calisthenics," for example.

Going outside to hike or take a walk is another important thing you should do, especially if you can get some sun while you're at it (for a natural source of vitamin D). Walking is a good choice and a highly underrated form of exercise.

The key is to choose something that you enjoy and can stick with in the long run.

If you're completely out of shape or have medical problems, it's a good idea to talk to your doctor or a qualified health professional before starting a new training program.

3. Sleep like a Baby

Sleep is very important for overall health and studies show that sleep deprivation correlates with many diseases, including obesity and heart disease (6Trusted Source, 7, 8Trusted Source).

It's highly recommended to make time for good, quality sleep. If you can't seem to sleep properly, there are several ways you can try to improve it:

- Don't drink coffee late in the day.

- Try to go to bed and wake up at similar times each day.

- Sleep in complete darkness, with no artificial lighting.

- Dim the lights in your home a few hours before bedtime.

- For more tips on how to improve your sleep, check out this article.

It may also be a good idea to see your doctor. Sleep disorders, such as sleep apnea, are very common and in many cases easily treatable.

4. Avoid Excess Stress

A healthy lifestyle involves a wholesome diet, quality sleep and regular exercise.

But the way you feel and how you think is also very important. Being stressed all the time is a recipe for disaster.

Excess stress can raise cortisol levels and severely impair your metabolism. It can increase junk food cravings, fat in your stomach area and raise your risk of various diseases.

Studies also show that stress is a significant contributor to depression, which is a massive health problem today.

To reduce stress, try to simplify your life — exercise, take nature walks, practice deep-breathing techniques and maybe even meditation.

If you absolutely cannot handle the burdens of your daily life without becoming overly stressed, consider seeing a psychologist.

Not only will overcoming your stress make you healthier, it will also improve your life in other ways. Going through life worried, anxious and never being able to relax and enjoy you is a big waste.

5. Nourish Your Body With Real Foods

The simplest and most effective way to eat healthy is to focus on real foods.

Choose unprocessed, whole foods that resemble what they looked like in nature.

It's best to eat a combination of animals and plants — meat, fish, eggs, vegetables, fruits, nuts, seeds, as well as healthy fats, oils and high-fat dairy products.

If you're healthy, lean and active, eating whole, unrefined carbs is absolutely fine. These include potatoes, sweet potatoes, legumes and whole grains such as oats.

However, if you're overweight, obese or have shown signs of metabolic issues such as diabetes or metabolic syndrome, then cutting back on major carbohydrate sources can lead to dramatic improvements.

People can often lose a lot of weight simply by cutting back on carbohydrates because they subconsciously start eating less.

Whatever you do, make an effort to choose whole, unprocessed foods instead of foods that look like they were made in a factory.

Things You Can Do for Your Health Today

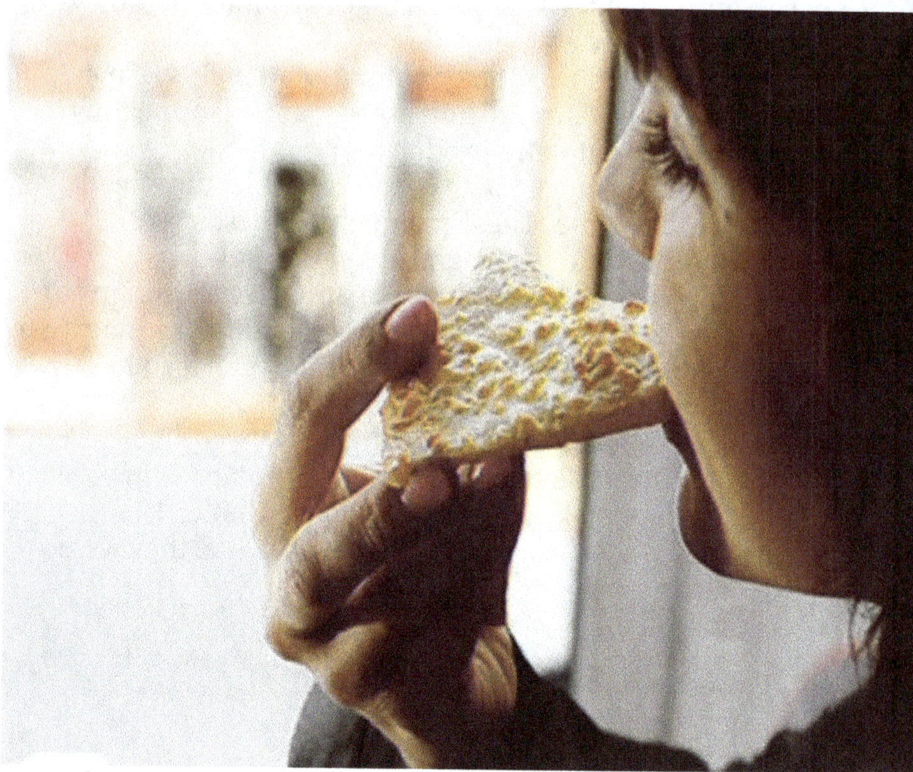

Eat Slowly

1/15

This gives your brain the chance to get the signal that you're full, so you're less likely to overeat. And if you take it slow, you're more likely to think about what you're eating and make sensible, healthy choices.

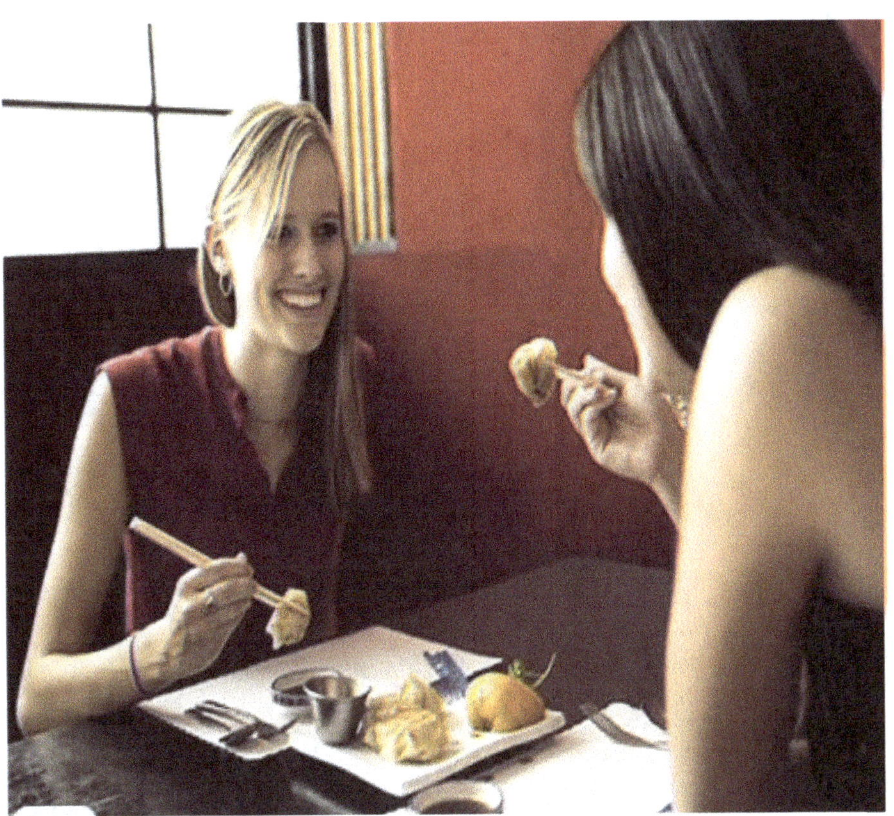

Socialize

2/15

It's not about how many people you know or how often you see them. What matters is a real connection with others. It can make you happier, more productive, and less likely to have health problems. So call up a friend and go to dinner or join a team or club to make some new ones.

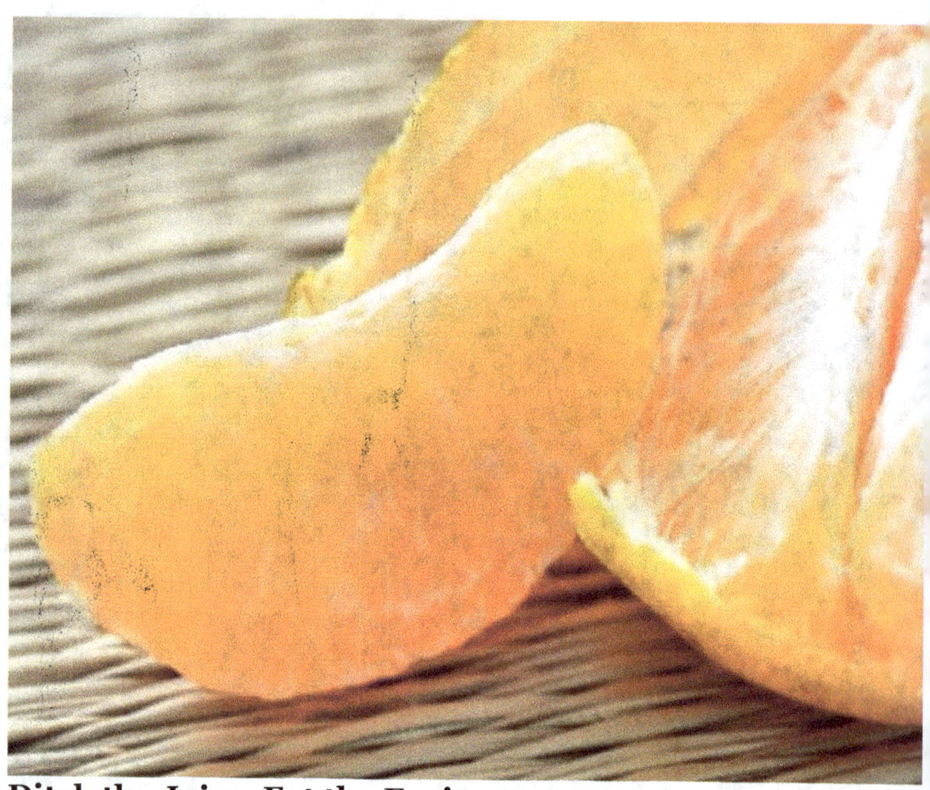

Ditch the Juice, Eat the Fruit

3/15

If you like orange juice, have an orange instead. Even 100% pure juice loses nutrition when you process it, and it can put a lot of hidden sugar in your diet. On the other hand, actual fruits are good sources of vitamin C, potassium, fiber, and folic acid. And they're low in fat, sodium, and calories.

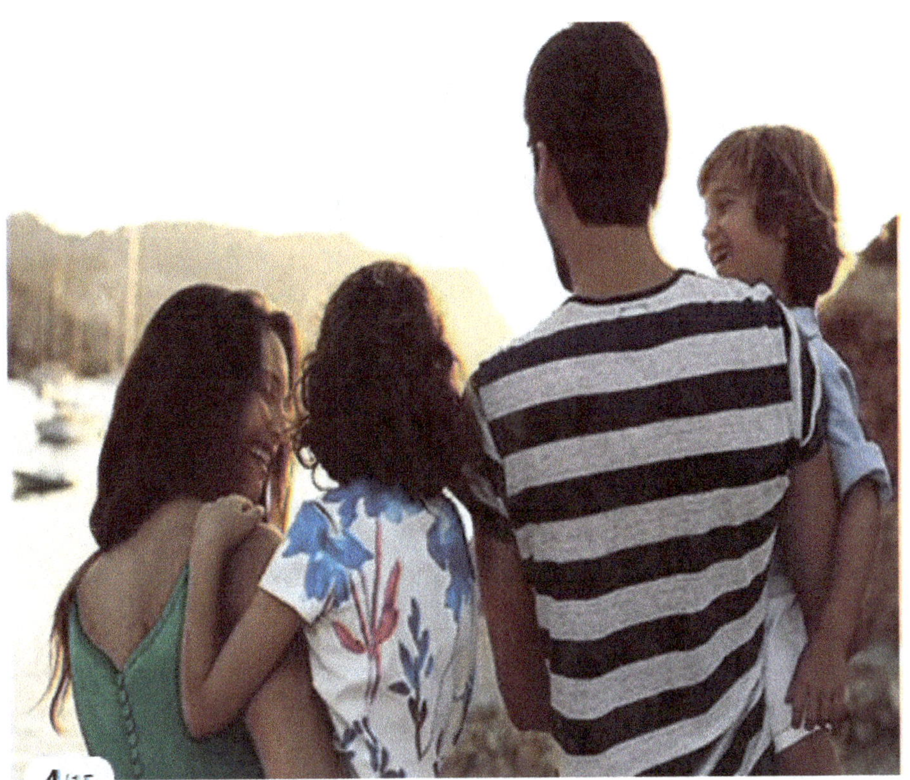

Take Time Off

4/15

It's a time when you can bond with family and friends, which is good for your mental and physical health. People who take more vacations live longer and are less likely to have heart disease and other health problems.

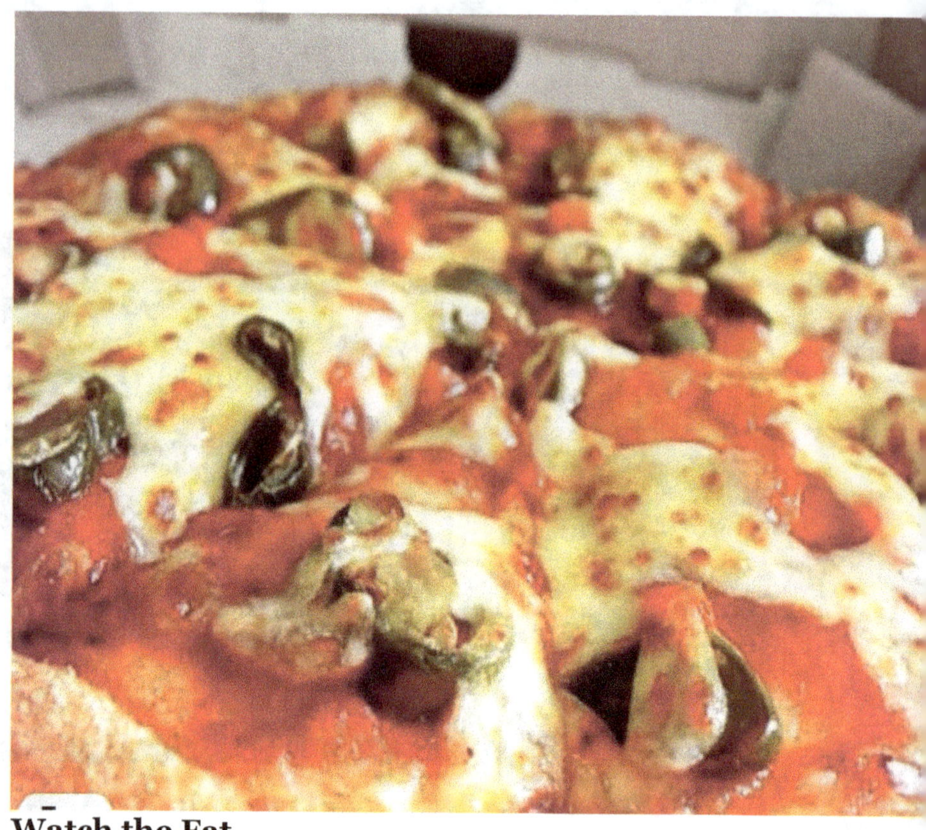

Watch the Fat

5/15

It's not as clear-cut as it sounds. You definitely want to keep an eye on trans fats, which are added to some foods (like frozen pizza and baked goods) to keep them fresh. They've been linked to heart disease. But some fat -- from dairy, whole eggs, fish, avocado, or nuts, for example -- is good for you as part of a balanced diet. And high-fat dairy may even help you lose weight better than low fat. This may be because the fat satisfies your hunger better than other calories.

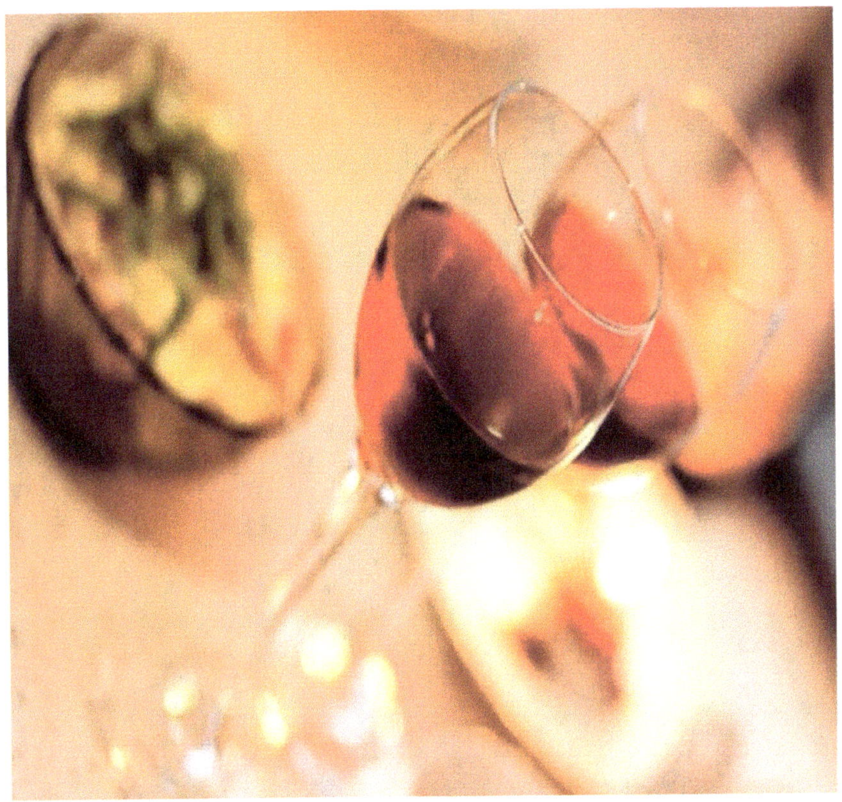

Have a Drink

6/15

Yes, we're talking about alcohol, but please notice the "a drink" part: two a day at most for men, one at most for women. More than that and the health benefits move quickly in the opposite direction. But a little alcohol can be good for your heart health, your stress level, and even your sex life.

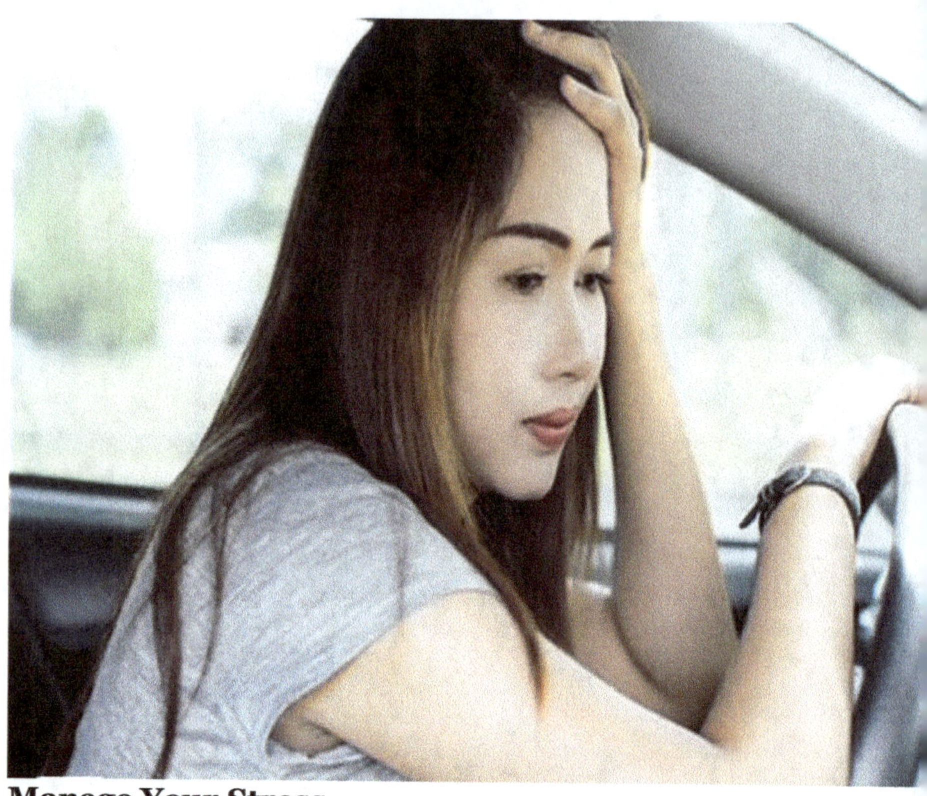

Manage Your Stress

7/15

We all have stress in our lives. It makes your muscles tense and your heart race. If this happens a lot -- during your daily commute, for example -- and you don't handle it well, it can cause serious health problems, including high blood pressure, ulcers, and heart disease. So take time to breathe, do something that calms you, and try to accept what you cannot change -- like rush-hour traffic.

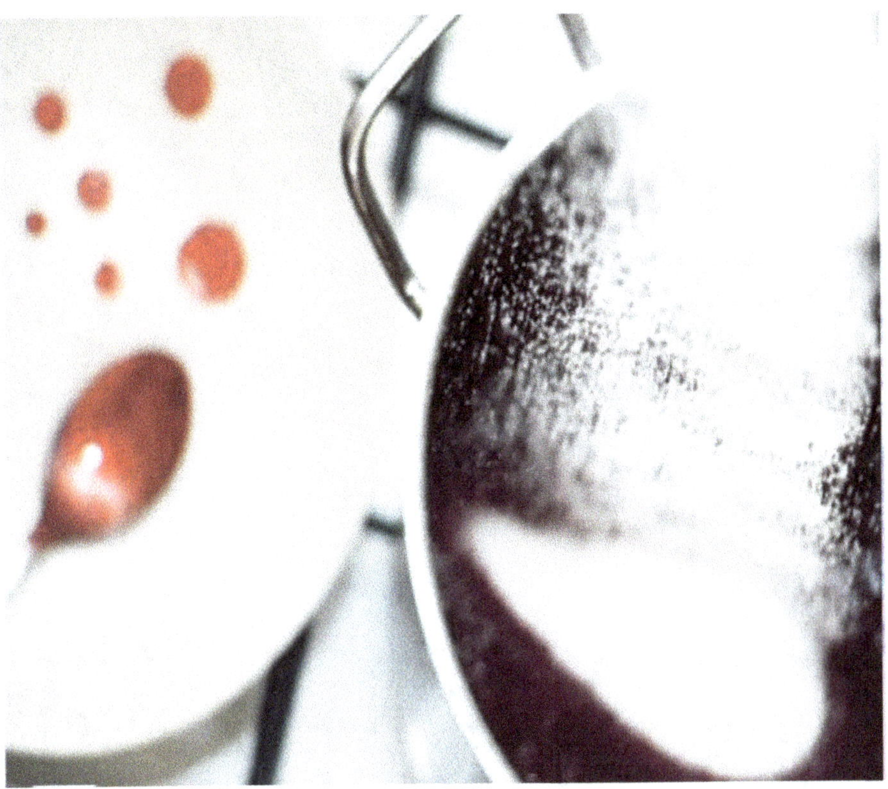

Cut Back on Sugar

8/15

Most of us get way more of it than we need. It's not just the added calories and the lack of nutritional value: It also can make your blood sugar spike and then crash, and that leaves you tired, hungry, and irritable -- "hangry."

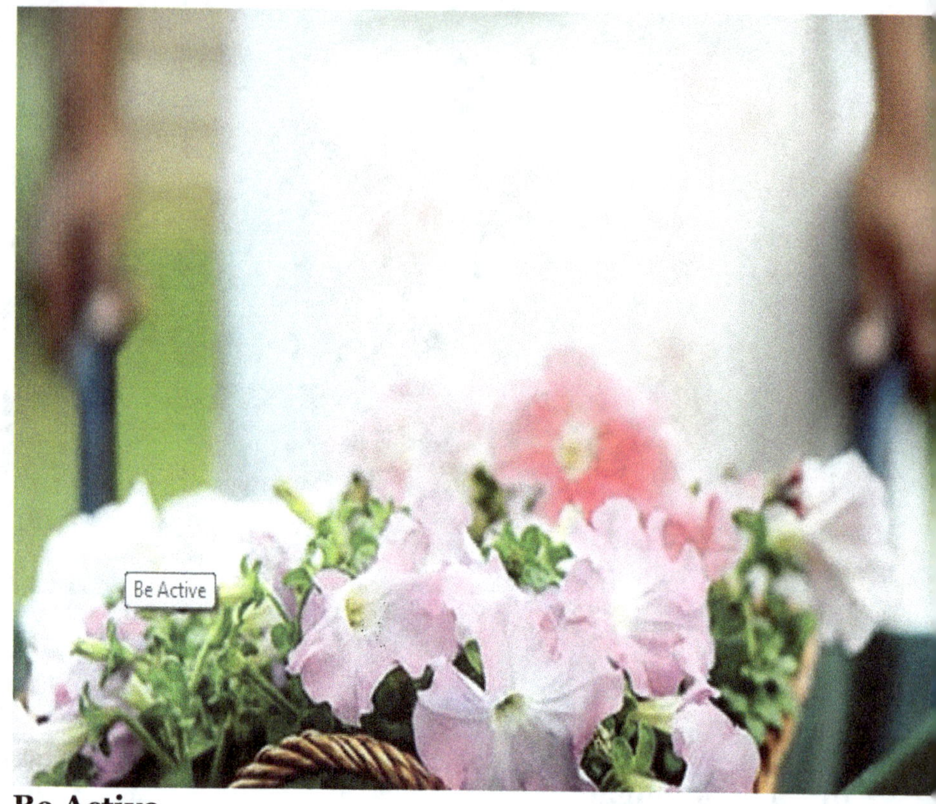

Be Active

9/15

Exercise is a proven way to improve your health, your mental well-being, and even your libido. You don't have to sign up for the New York Marathon -- just get your heart rate up for 30 minutes or so a few times a week. Gardening works, and so does a walk around the block. If you can't make it a habit on your own, try to make it social: Join a local sports league or plan regular runs with a friend.

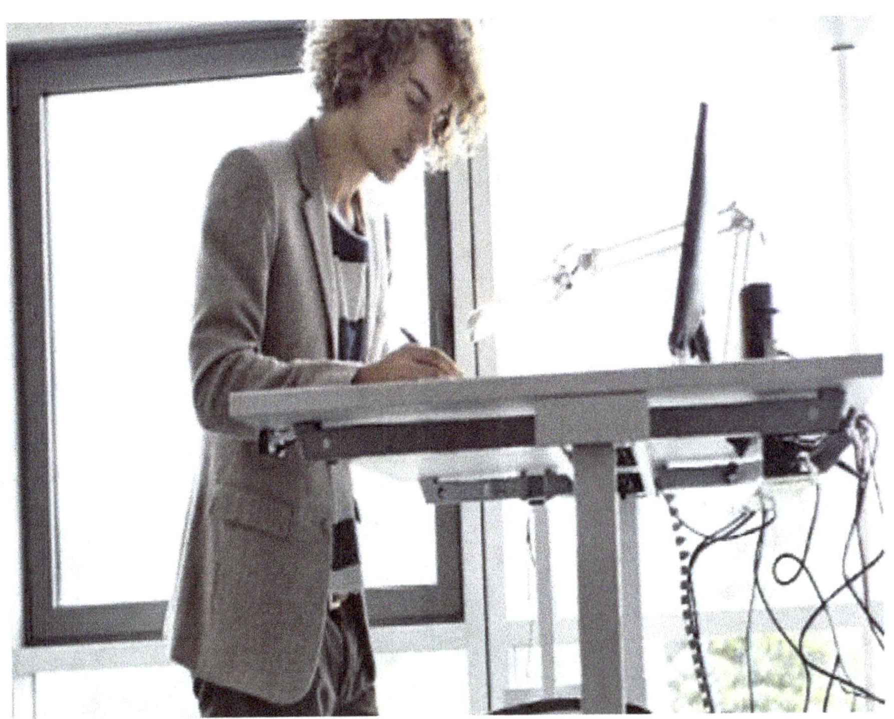

Keep Moving

10/15

If you work in an office, get up and walk around every hour or so, or try a standing desk for part of the day. You'll burn more calories, improve your circulation, and stay more alert. It may even help prevent certain health issues, like diabetes and high blood pressure.

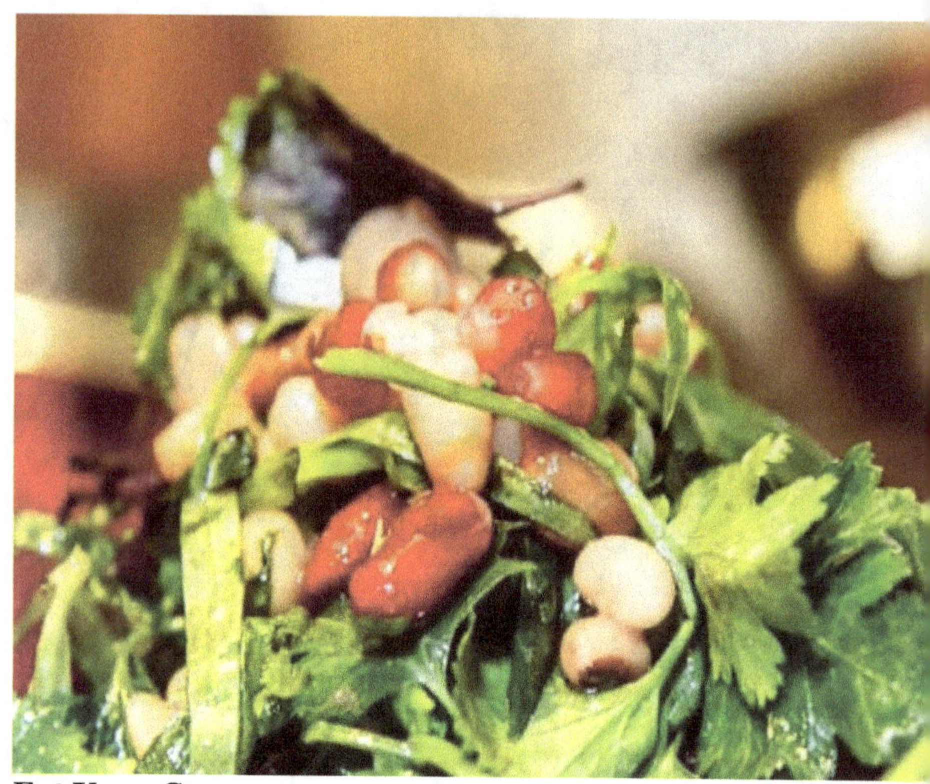

Eat Your Greens

11/15

Kale, spinach, collards, Romaine, arugula, Bok choy, broccolini -- make sure you get plenty of these leafy green vegetables. They're chock full of nutrients, low in calories, and have loads of fiber, which fills you up and satisfies your hunger.

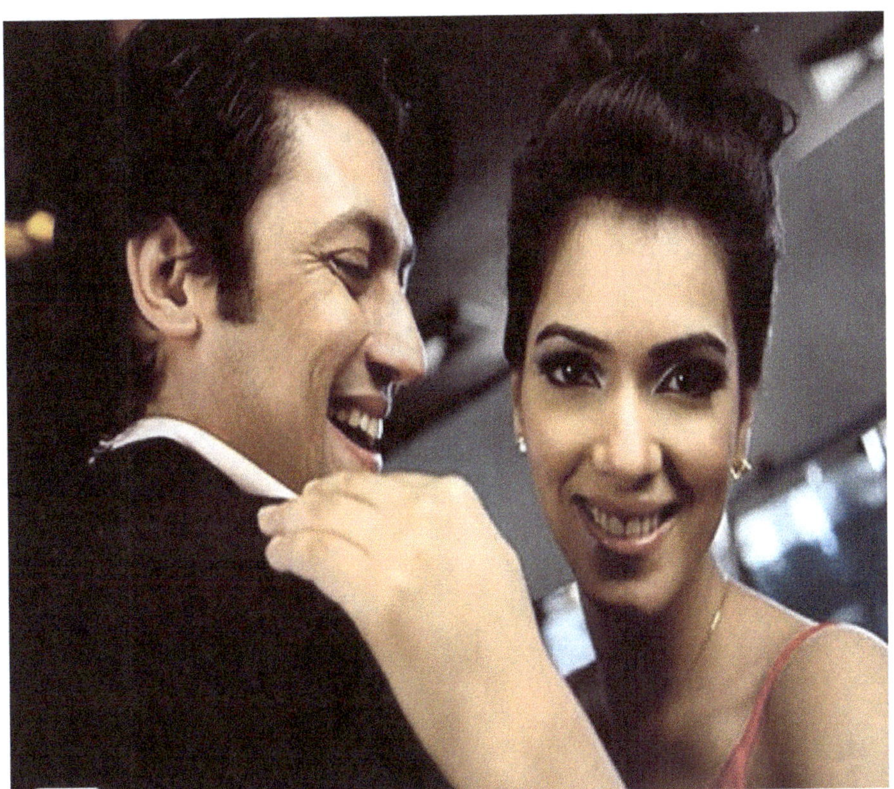

Dance

12/15

It keeps your mind sharp because it's a skill that involves body movement, and that's especially good for your brain. It's also social and can be lots of fun, which bring health benefits of their own. And you might not even notice that you're exercising!

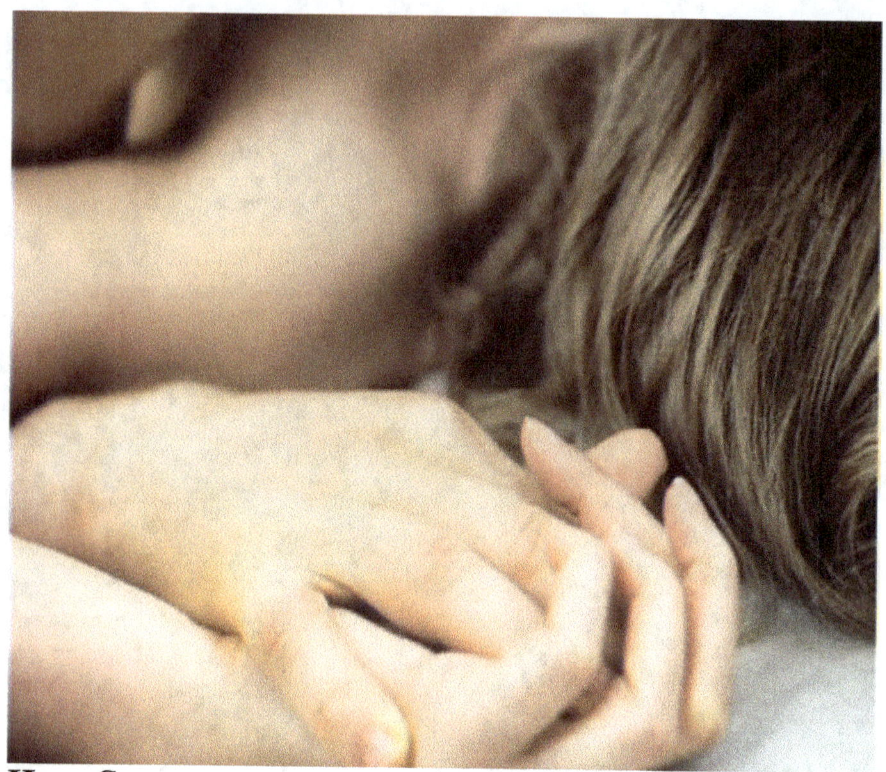

Have Sex

13/15

It's linked to heart health, brain health, a long life, a strong relationship, and even happiness. Just keep it safe. Get tested for STDs and use condoms to protect yourself and your partner against diseases and unwanted pregnancy.

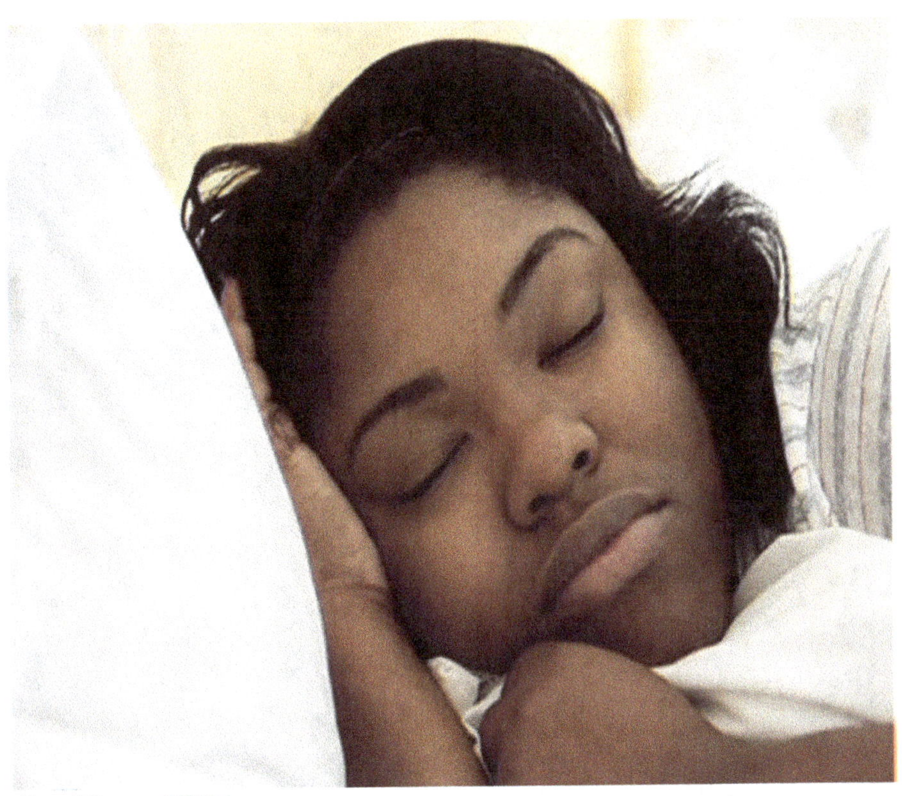

Get Your ZZZs

14/15

A lack of sleep can lead to diabetes, heart disease, obesity, and depression. If that's not enough reason to get your ZZZs, it also causes car crashes and other accidents. Adults should get 7 to 9 hours each night.

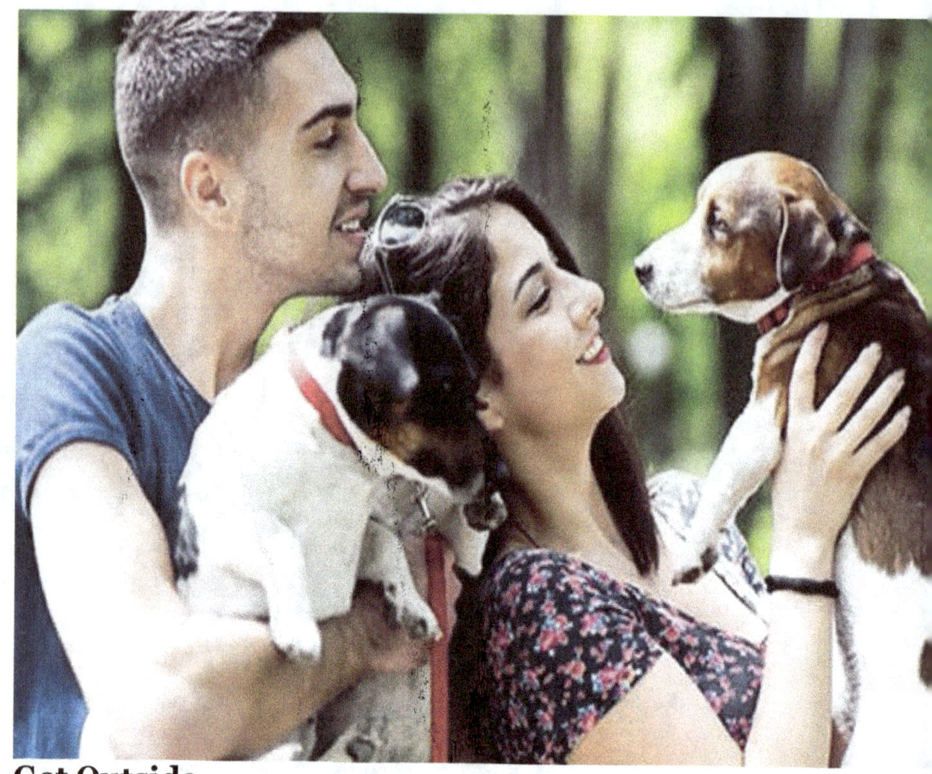

Get Outside

15/15

The sunlight helps set your sleep clock and leads to more exercise. You'll also get vitamin D, which many people don't get enough of. It's important for cell function, mental health, and heart health. But don't stay in the sun too long, and wear sunscreen. Too much sun is linked to skin cancer.

Amazing Ways to Improve Your Health in One Day

Every once in a while, eating fast food, getting a poor night's sleep, and skipping a workout isn't a huge deal. But when these become increasingly frequent habits, you're bound to end up feeling pretty lousy. When you get to that place, it can seem impossible to turn things around and get back to your healthy, vibrant self again. The good news is, it's easier than you think—in fact, you can improve your health in as few as 24 hours.

Woman exercising early in the morning

Shutter stock

Every once in a while, eating fast food, getting a poor night's sleep, and skipping a workout isn't a huge deal. But when these become increasingly frequent habits, you're bound to end up feeling pretty lousy. When you get to that place, it can seem impossible to turn things around and get back to your healthy, vibrant self again. The good news is, it's easier than you think—in fact, you can improve your health in as few as 24 hours.

1. Don't wait so long to eat breakfast.

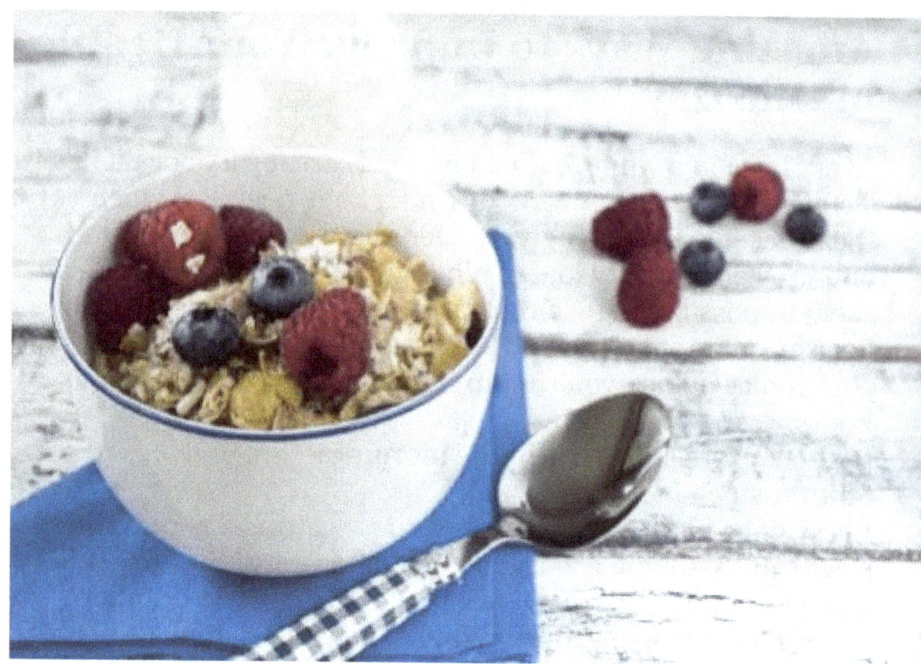

Intermittent fasting may have been a trend, but in order to improve your health quickly, you'll want to eat breakfast. "Be sure to eat within one hour of waking up," says Cara Clark, CN, a California-based certified nutritionist and owner of Cara Clark Nutrition. "If you aren't eating first thing in the morning after fasting overnight, then you're keeping a slower metabolism and low blood sugar, potentially even causing your body to store fat when you do finally eat." And for more reasons why you should eat something with your morning coffee, check out Skipping Breakfast Can Significantly Shorten Your Lifespan, Study Says.

2. And start your day with warm lemon water.

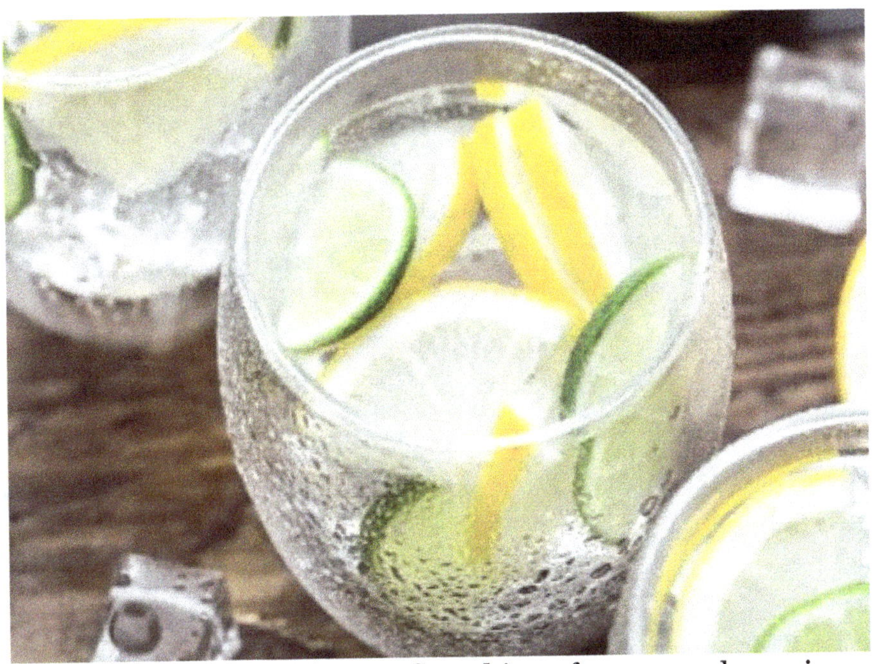

Drinking a big glass of water first thing after you wake up is one of the most refreshing things you can do in the morning. But the next time you do so, add some lemon for extra health-boosting benefits. "Start each morning with warm lemon water," says Robyn Yokels, a certified health coach in New York and Los Angeles, and author of Go With Your Gut. "It's one of the oldest tricks in the book, but that's because it works."

According to Yokels, it's "a gentle way to wake up your digestive system and can help support your body's natural detox systems, reducing puffiness and bloating." If you want to give yourself an extra boost, "you can also add lemon to your water throughout the day," she says. And for more ways to start your day off right, check out these 50 Inspirational Morning Quotes to Kick Off Your Day.

3. Avoid processed foods.

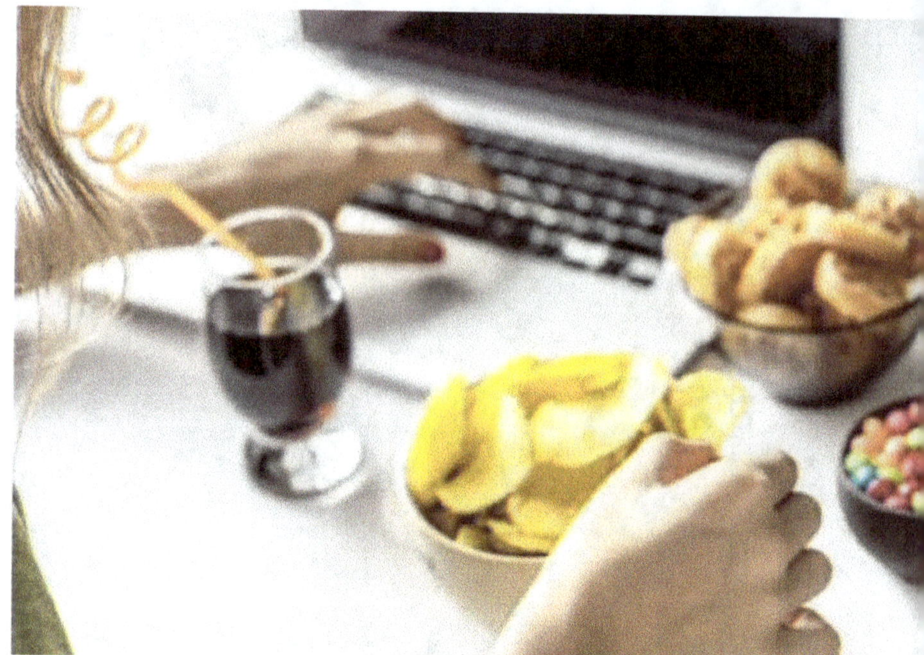

We know processed foods taste delicious, but unfortunately, most of them won't do anything for you but make you feel lethargic. "Eating a standard American diet containing loads of added salt, sugar, and fat can lead to symptoms of depression and anxiety, while eating real, unprocessed foods—like nuts, veggies, fruit, and whole grains—will keep your mood up and give you natural energy," says Hilary Hinrichs, a certified health coach and owner of Holistic Hilary in New York City.

4. Cut back on sodium.

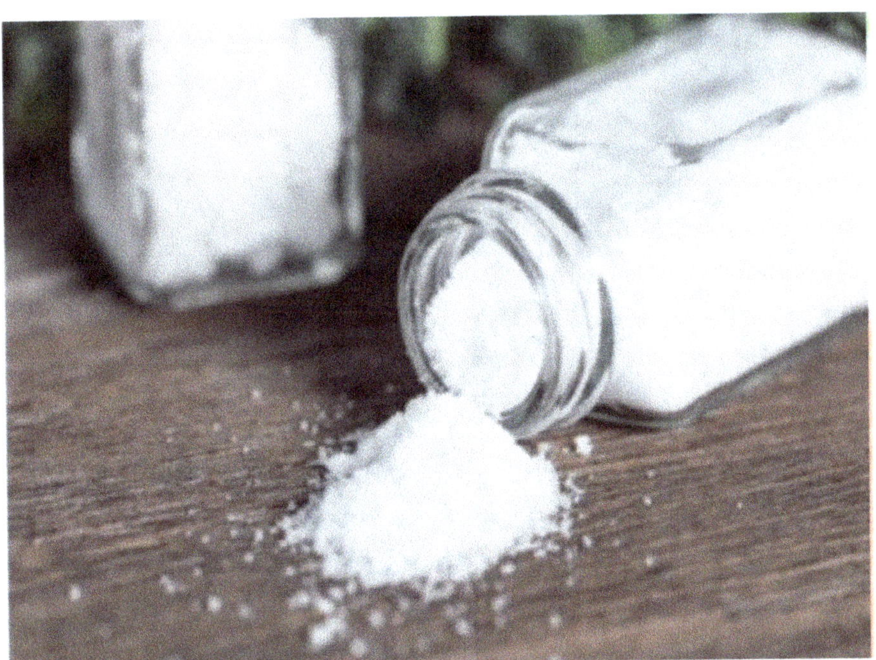

Sodium is everywhere. And when you're eating too much of it, you're going to feel the not-so-fun effects. "When you take in a lot of sodium, you can feel bloated and inflamed," says Gorin. "Sodium can sneak into many foods—especially packaged foods, including frozen meals. Even bread can be a problem." The American Heart Association recommends no more than 2,300 milligrams of sodium a day and moving toward an ideal limit of no more than 1,500 milligrams a day for most adults. "When you decrease your salt intake, you can immediately feel less bloated and healthier," says Gorin. And for the foods you should be eating instead, try some of the 33 Foods That Fight Aging from the Inside Out.

5. Drink your fruit and veggies.

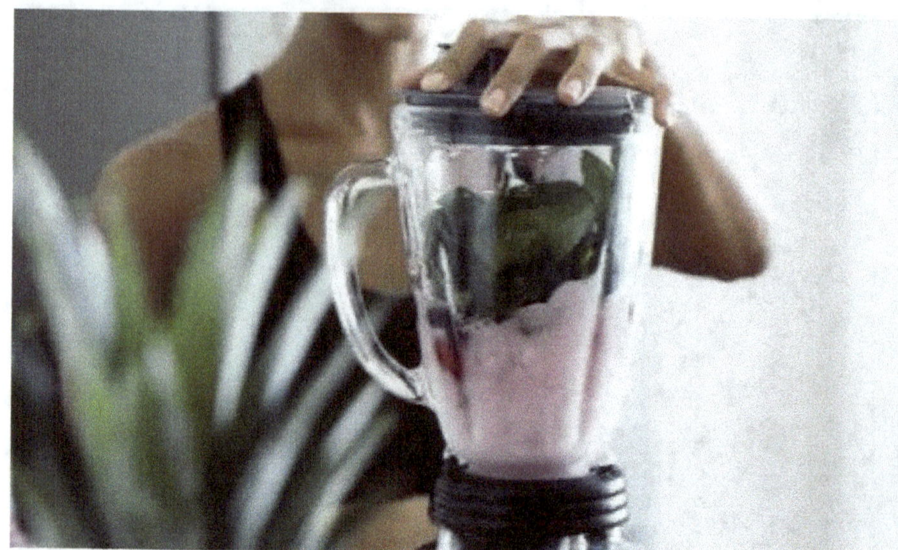

You aren't just limited to eating your fruits and veggies. Gorin says it's important to remember that you can drink them, too. "One of the easiest ways to help your health is to include vegetables or fruit with every meal or snack. That not only means fresh fruits and veggies, but also 100 percent juice," she says. "Getting your daily servings of produce in the short-term may help lower blood pressure, digestion, and hydration. Then in the long-term, it helps lower your risk of heart disease and certain types of cancer."

6. Rethink where you get your fluids.

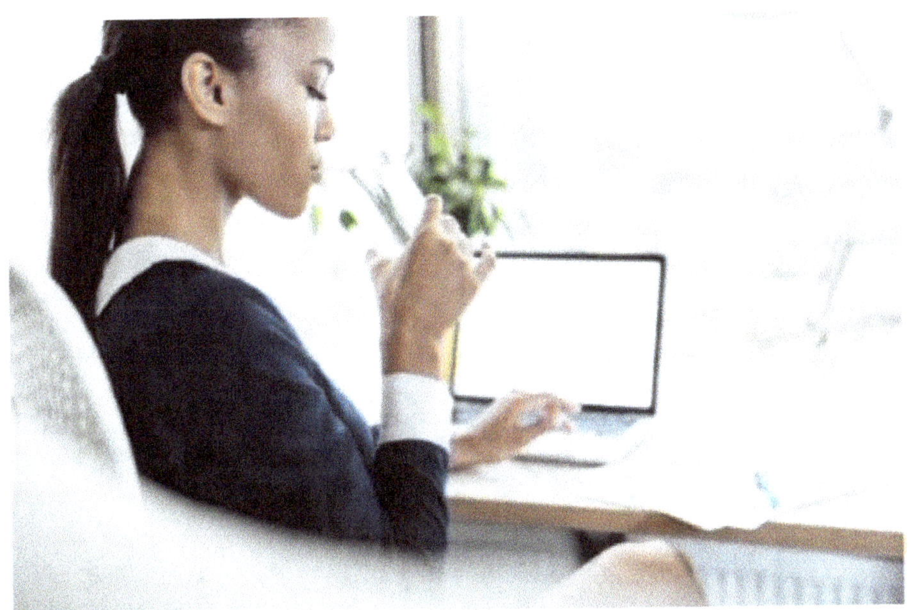

You might feel like you're perfectly hydrated. But when you think about it, how much water are you actually drinking? "The number one method you can use to turn your health around in one day is increasing your water intake," says Jenny Carr, a Wyoming-based certified anti-inflammatory health coach and author of Peace of Cake: The Secret to an Anti-Inflammatory Diet. "Pure, clean water detoxifies, stabilizes blood sugar levels, lubricates joints, and—of course—hydrates," she says.

7. And carry around a water bottle.

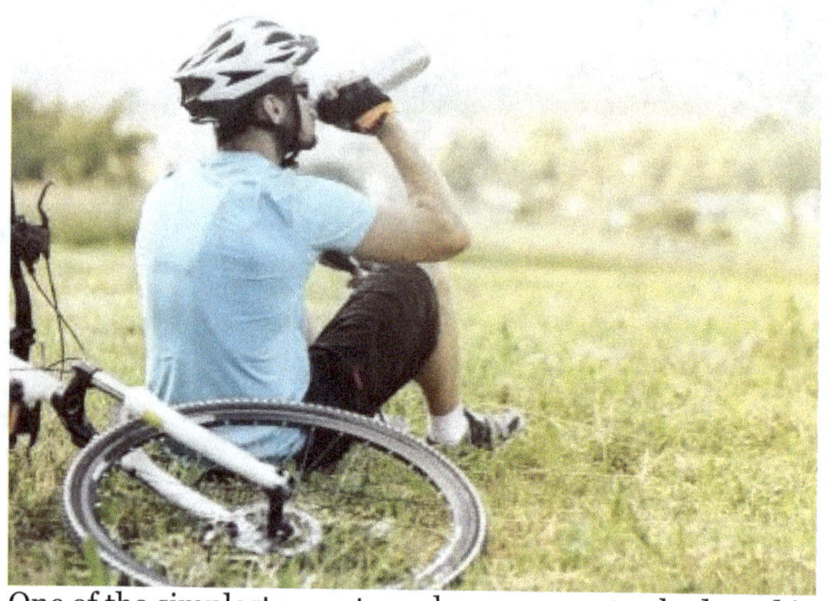

One of the simplest ways to make sure you stay hydrated is to carry a water bottle wherever you go.

"Drinking enough water and being properly hydrated can impact your health in so many ways, from decreasing your headaches to helping relieve constipation," Gorin says. "Carry a water bottle around with you during the day, and sip often. And don't forget to drink up at meals! If you're not a water fan, unsweetened tea can also help hydrate you." And for some chic water bottle options, try one of the 25 Cute Water Bottles That Will Keep You Hydrated All Summer.

8. Stretch it out.

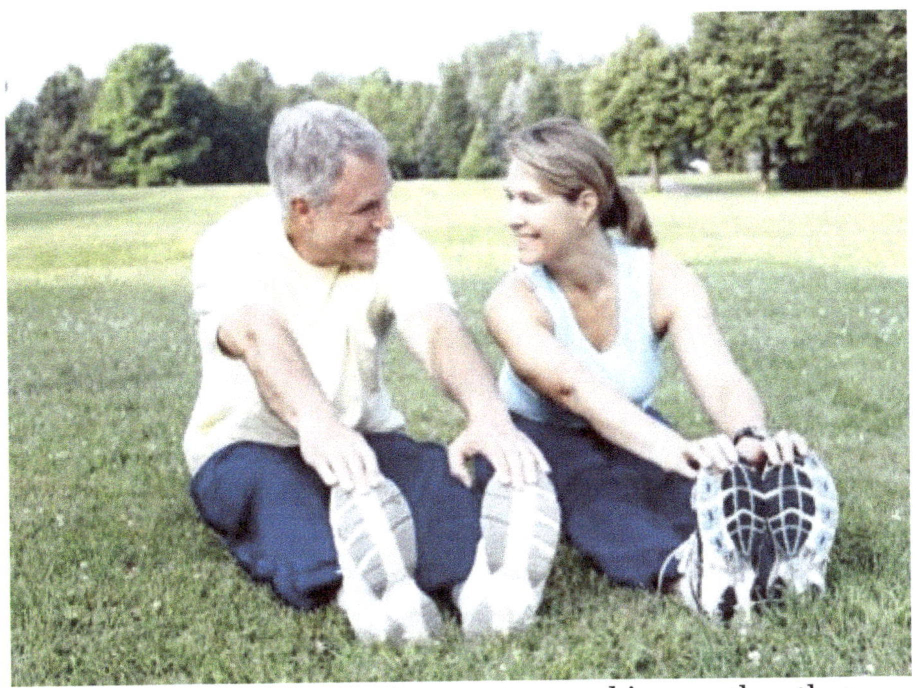

You know that working out is a must; stretching, on the other hand, sometimes gets brushed aside. Not only does stretching make you feel better in the moment, but according to Harvard Medical School, it also keeps you flexible, strong, and mobile as you age. Additionally, it's a quick and effective way to combat the tension in your body that can cause headaches, neck pain, jaw pain, and more.

9. Go for a triple-threat meal combo.

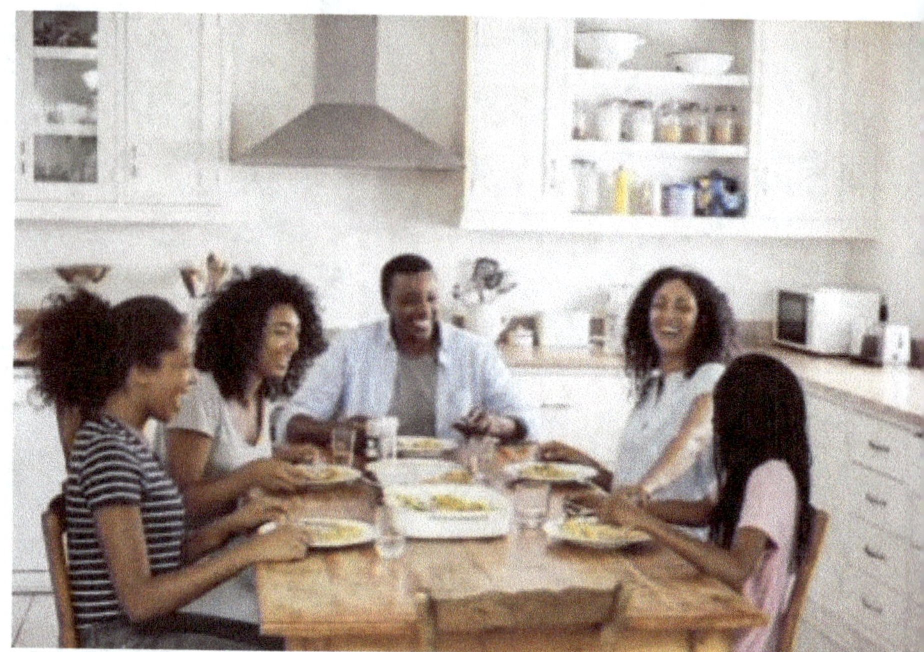

There's no longer any need to wonder what to put on your plate to help you feel your best. According to Clark, you can keep it simple by focusing on three key groups that will help improve your health today and in the future. "Combine a lean protein, healthy fat, and carbohydrate in every meal," she says. "This will lead to optimal energy and fat burning." And for even more ways to boost your energy, try these 25 Ways to Boost Your Energy Level Without Coffee.

10. Do some deep breathing exercises.

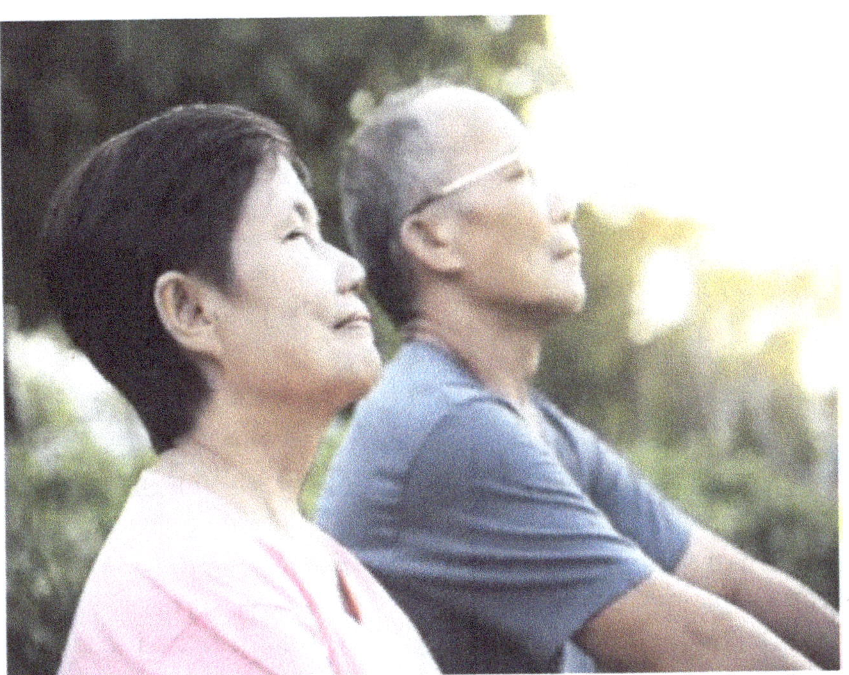

How often do you take the time to really breathe during the day? Not short, shallow, stressed-out breaths, but deep ins and outs that instantly energize you? According to Harvard Medical School, deep breathing—also known as diaphragmatic breathing—results in a full oxygen exchange in your body that can slow your heartbeat and keep your blood pressure in check, not to mention help ease tension and anxiety.

"We often go about our busy days without checking in on ourselves to see how we're feeling," says Hendricks. "Taking deep breaths every hour can help combat stress and make you feel happier and more content to carry on with your day." And for more ways to improve your heart health, avoid the 27 Daily Habits That Are Ruining Your Heart.

11. Make sure you're reading nutrition labels.

Don't just grab something from the shelf and put it in your cart. Before you decide to buy an item at the grocery store, Gorin says to make sure you're reading the nutrition label first. Many of the items on store shelves contain a lot of sodium and added sugar—two things that can keep you from feeling your best. Once you cut them out, your health will start improving immediately.

12. Switch up the way you get your protein.

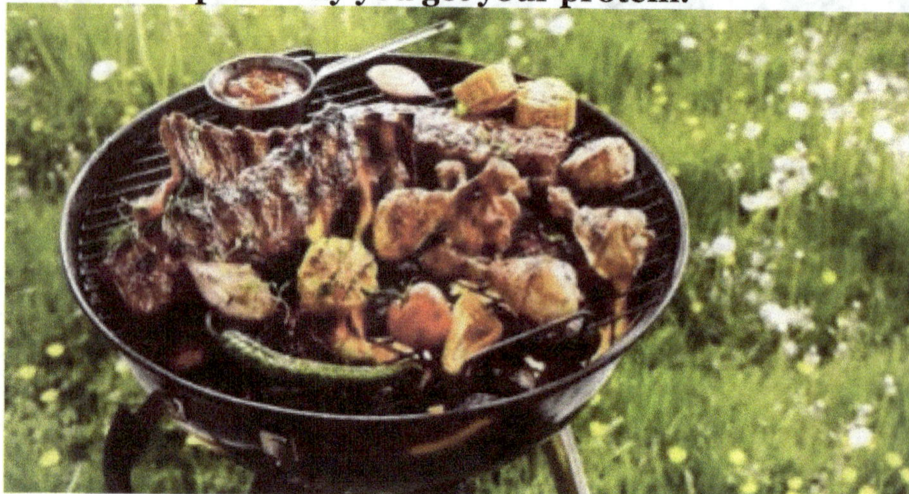

A protein deficiency probably isn't something you need to worry about: According to Harvard Health, most American adults consume more than enough. The real thing to focus on for better health is which kind you're eating.

"Very often when we're feeling low-energy, nauseous, or have a difficult time focusing, it's because our blood sugar levels are out of whack," Carr explains. "Eating clean protein—meaning organic, plant-based protein with no fillers, or grass-fed, free-range, or wild-caught meat—is a quick way to ground you and stabilize your blood sugar levels." And if you're still feeling low energy, it could be one of the 45 Sneaky Signs you're Unhealthier than You May Think.

AUTHORS NAME: Curtis H. Ledbetter
CONTACT INFO: curtish.ledbetterauthor@gmail.com

www.ingramcontent.com/pod-product-compliance
Lightning Source LLC
Chambersburg PA
CBHW060058260726
48658CB00004B/1331